Psychopharmacology:

501 Questions to Help You Pass the Boards

Vithyalakshmi Selvaraj, MD

Staff Psychiatrist
Department of Veterans Affairs
Instructor in Psychiatry
Creighton University School of Medicine
Omaha, Nebraska

Sriram Ramaswamy, MD

Staff Psychiatrist
Department of Veterans Affairs
Associate Chair for Research
Associate Professor of Psychiatry
Creighton University School of Medicine
Omaha, Nebraska

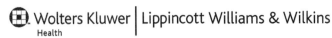
Wolters Kluwer | Lippincott Williams & Wilkins
Health

Philadelphia • Baltimore • New York • London
Buenos Aires • Hong Kong • Sydney • Tokyo

Acquisitions Editor: Julie Goolsby
Product Manager: Tom Gibbons
Vendor Manager: Bridgett Dougherty
Senior Manufacturing Manager: Benjamin Rivera
Marketing Manager: Alexander Burns
Design Coordinator: Holly McLaughlin
Production Service: S4Carlisle

Printed in China

Library of Congress Cataloging-in-Publication Data
[978-1-4511-1692-2]
[1-4511-1692-6]
Selvaraj, Vithyalakshmi, 1977-
  Psychopharmacology : 501 questions to help you pass the boards / Vithyalakshmi Selvaraj, Sriram Ramaswamy.
    p. ; cm.
  Includes bibliographical references and index.
  ISBN 978-1-4511-1692-2 (alk. paper) — ISBN 1-4511-1692-6 (alk. paper)
  I. Ramaswamy, Sriram, 1972- II. Title.
  [DNLM: 1. Psychotropic Drugs—pharmacology—Examination Questions. 2. Psychopharmacology—methods—Examination Questions. 3. Psychotropic Drugs—therapeutic use—Examination Questions. QV 18.2]

  615.7'88—dc23

                                2012009480

Care has been taken to confirm the accuracy of the information presented and to describe generally accepted practices. However, the authors, editors, and publisher are not responsible for errors or omissions or for any consequences from application of the information in this book and make no warranty, expressed or implied, with respect to the currency, completeness, or accuracy of the contents of the publication. Application of the information in a particular situation remains the professional responsibility of the practitioner.

The authors, editors, and publisher have exerted every effort to ensure that drug selection and dosage set forth in this text are in accordance with current recommendations and practice at the time of publication. However, in view of ongoing research, changes in government regulations, and the constant flow of information relating to drug therapy and drug reactions, the reader is urged to check the package insert for each drug for any change in indications and dosage and for added warnings and precautions. This is particularly important when the recommended agent is a new or infrequently employed drug.

Some drugs and medical devices presented in the publication have Food and Drug Administration (FDA) clearance for limited use in restricted research settings. It is the responsibility of the health care provider to ascertain the FDA status of each drug or device planned for use in their clinical practice.

To purchase additional copies of this book, call our customer service department at (800) 638-3030 or fax orders to (301) 223-2320. International customers should call (301) 223-2300.

Visit Lippincott Williams & Wilkins on the Internet: at LWW.com. Lippincott Williams & Wilkins customer service representatives are available from 8:30 am to 6 pm, EST.

10 9 8 7 6 5 4 3 2 1

We would like to dedicate this wealth of knowledge to our daughters—Nila Chandramouli and Nikita, and Tanya Ramaswamy.

Contents

FOREWORD

The practice of psychiatry and the principles of psychopharmacologic treatment are amid much transformation with great challenges ahead. The proliferation of biologic and psychopharmacologic science coupled with an emphasis on evidenced-based and cost-effective care makes it difficult for clinicians to continuously integrate current information into daily practice. Moreover, there is an unmet need for resources to train the next generation of psychiatrists and psychopharmacologists. Psychiatrists, mental health nurse practitioners, and other psychiatric providers especially need means to further develop their skills and competence in psychopharmacology. Thus, it is timely and of great importance that a clear and practical yet truly expert book focusing solely on principles and practice of psychopharmacology and with ABPN-style questions for self-assessment is finally available. With this, Drs. Selvaraj and Ramaswamy offer adroit assistance to anyone interested in assuring competence in contemporary psychopharmacology.

Dr. Vithya Selvaraj, the primary author, is a rapidly rising junior colleague with a strong psychopharmacology knowledge and an expanding research portfolio. During her psychiatric training in the United Kingdom, she created a database of extended multiple choice questions to help physicians prepare for the Professional and Linguistic Assessments Board (PLAB) test. The PLAB test is the main route by which International Medical Graduates demonstrate they have the necessary skills and knowledge to practice medicine in the United Kingdom. As a pioneer in the Primary Care-Mental Health Integration program within the Department of Veterans Affairs, Vithya is also well versed with the psychopharmacology needs of primary care physicians. Such expertise makes this book an extremely useful resource for the growing number of primary care doctors and other practitioners prescribing psychotropic medications.

Dr. Sriram Ramaswamy is yet another superb faculty member whom I have personally known for the past 10 years. Dr. Ramaswamy has an excellent academic track record based on psychiatric training and clinical experience both in India and in the United States. Currently, he directs the Creighton Psychopharmacology Research program and also practices in various clinical settings—community clinics, Veterans Affairs, correctional care, and so on. He is well published. Again, such expertise assures that this book is both practical and precise.

Having known both authors well for many years, I am not at all surprised that they have achieved a remarkable feat in the creation of more than 500 board exam–style questions with clear and accurate explanations that encompass the full spectrum of psychopharmacologic treatments across all age groups and comorbidities! From my personal experience as writer and editor for the exam questions, I can testify that this book is an extraordinary achievement that integrates the authors' clinical experiences with current evidence-based data. Readers of this book will not put it on the shelf but will scour it from cover to cover.

Daniel R. Wilson, MD, PhD

Vice-President for Health Affairs and Dean of Medicine
Professor of Psychiatry, Neurology and Anthropology
University of Florida
Jacksonville, Florida

PREFACE

We proudly present the first edition of our book *Psychopharmacology: 501 Questions to Help You Pass the Boards*! We decided to write this book for several reasons. Psychopharmacology is a rapidly expanding field. Given the recent changes in the delivery of mental health care, more nonpsychiatrists (primary care physicians, psychologists, psychiatric nurse practitioners, and physician assistants) are being called upon to prescribe psychiatric medications. These changes have created a need and demand for specific psychopharmacology training programs and courses. Furthermore, psychiatric residents and board-eligible as well as board-certified psychiatrists are required to pass exams such as the annual Psychiatry Resident-In-Training Examination, American Board of Psychiatry and Neurology board certification, and Maintenance of Certification exams. In all, this has created an unmet need for board review materials in psychopharmacology.

Our book has five chapters with ABPN board–style questions to help you prepare and breeze through the boards. It covers all topics in clinical psychopharmacology. In addition to testing current treatment options and trends, older-generation and often neglected yet clinically valuable psychotropic agents are covered. The multiple-choice format will make the experience more enjoyable and increase the interest in the topic at hand. Also, readers will be able to reflect on the correct as well as wrong answers, making learning subsequent material more efficient. The intended audience for this book is psychiatric residents, practicing psychiatrists, licensed psychologists, advanced practice nurses, nurse practitioners, physician's assistants, and pharmacists.

The questions are evidence based and also drawn from our own personal prescribing experience. We encourage readers to cross-check treatment recommendations and doses with standard reference textbooks. We have questions based on clinically relevant data from pivotal psychiatric clinical studies such as CATIE, STAR-D, and so on.

There are so many people to thank in writing this book. We would like to profusely thank our mentors—Drs. Daniel R. Wilson, Subhash C. Bhatia, and Frederick Petty—for their steady support towards our scholarly pursuits. We are eternally indebted to their wisdom and unwavering confidence in our abilities. We would like to thank our families for their support and motivation.

We thank the editors at Lippincott Williams & Wilkins for their helpful suggestions. We are indebted to our patients whom we have treated over the years. We have learnt so much from them as partners in their journey to mental health recovery.

Acknowledgment

This material is the result of work supported with resources and the use of facilities at the VA Nebraska-Western Iowa Health Care System.

Chapter 1

Adult Psychopharmacology

Questions

1. Which of the following medications can be safely used in combination with monoamine oxidase inhibitors (MAOIs)?

    A. Escitalopram

    B. Amitriptyline

    C. Meperidine

    D. Desvenlafaxine

    E. Bupropion

2. After discontinuation of an MAOI, endogenous monoamine oxidase (MAO) activity levels return to baseline levels after

    A. 1 week

    B. 2 weeks

    C. 3 weeks

    D. 4 weeks

    E. 6 weeks

3. A 36-year-old white woman who was involved in a motor vehicle accident about a year ago comes in complaining of recurrent intrusive recollections of the accident, experiences frequent flashbacks, avoids driving, and reports being emotionally detached from family and friends. On further questioning, she admits to frequent insomnia, nightmares, depressed mood, and an exaggerated startle response. Which of the following medications could potentially alleviate her symptoms by primarily antagonizing central presynaptic α_2-adrenergic receptors?

   A. Clonidine

   B. Mirtazapine

   C. Prazosin

   D. Venlafaxine

   E. Naltrexone

4. Which of the following is a common side effect of mirtazapine?

   A. Hypotension

   B. Weight gain

   C. Hyponatremia

   D. Liver toxicity

   E. Agranulocytosis

5. Which of the following statements is/are true regarding clozapine?

   A. Clozapine improves negative symptoms in schizophrenia

   B. Clozapine is effective in the management of treatment refractory bipolar depression

   C. Clozapine is not associated with the development of neuroleptic malignant syndrome (NMS)

   D. The incidence of clozapine-induced agranulocytosis is about 5%

   E. All of the above

6. The following antidepressants suppress rapid eye movement (REM) sleep EXCEPT:

    A. Bupropion

    B. Paroxetine

    C. Nortriptyline

    D. Fluoxetine

    E. Venlafaxine

7. Which of the following antipsychotics has the lowest risk of weight gain as a side effect after treatment?

    A. Aripiprazole

    B. Ziprasidone

    C. Quetiapine

    D. Molindone

    E. Paliperidone

8. All of the following drugs are associated with drug-induced depression EXCEPT:

    A. Alprazolam

    B. α-Interferon

    C. Propranolol

    D. Varenicline

    E. Depot-medroxyprogesterone acetate

9. All of the following are components of Sternbach criteria for the diagnosis of serotonin syndrome EXCEPT:

A. Myoclonus

B. Hyporeflexia

C. Diarrhea

D. Shivering

E. Fever

10. Which of the following statements regarding amoxapine is true?

A. Amoxapine is a norepinephrine reuptake inhibitor

B. Amoxapine can cause extrapyramidal side effects

C. Amoxapine is useful in the treatment of psychotic depression

D. Amoxapine overdose produces seizures

E. All of the above

11. Which of the following antipsychotic medications is least likely to cause orthostatic hypotension?

A. Fluphenazine

B. Thioridazine

C. Clozapine

D. Chlorpromazine

E. Olanzapine

12. A 45-year-old patient with bipolar disorder on lithium therapy presents with hair loss along with other constitutional symptoms. Which of the following is the most appropriate next step?

    A. Discontinue lithium and start another mood stabilizer

    B. Order a thyroid-stimulating hormone (TSH) level

    C. Prescribe selenium supplements

    D. Recommend a drug holiday to see if hair regrows

    E. None of the above

13. Ms. B, a 32-year-old woman, is seen for concerns regarding her appearance. She is referred to you by her primary care physician (PCP). The patient feels that her nose is misshapen and too large and her eyes are too far apart. She spends a significant amount of time camouflaging her face with makeup. The patient has had several consultations with specialists who have not found any abnormality at all. The patient requested her PCP for a referral to an aesthetic surgeon; however, her PCP wanted her to get a psychiatric evaluation first. After taking to her, you feel that she is quite preoccupied and delusional about her perceived defect. She is very anxious about this problem and has even quit her job trying to get this resolved. She denies any suicide thoughts or hallucinations. Which of the following agents would be the most appropriate choice for her condition?

    A. Aripiprazole

    B. Bupropion

    C. Amoxapine

    D. Fluoxetine

    E. Haloperidol

14. Which of the following drugs is contraindicated in patients with a history of allergy to tricyclic antidepressants (TCAs)?

    A. Carbamazepine

    B. Mirtazapine

    C. Trifluoperazine

    D. Lamotrigine

    E. Olanzapine

15. A 45-year-old man with treatment-resistant schizophrenia is started on clozapine. After 12 weeks of treatment with clozapine, his symptoms improve. However, his most recent WBC count is 1,800 per mm^3, and his absolute neutrophil count (ANC) is 900 per mm^3. What is the most appropriate next step?

    A. Taper clozapine over 7 days and monitor his WBC and ANC for an additional 2 weeks

    B. Discontinue clozapine immediately and monitor WBC and ANC for 4 weeks

    C. Continue clozapine but obtain daily blood cell counts until WBC count is >3,000 per mm^3 and ANC is >1,500 per mm^3

    D. Continue clozapine and request an hematology consult

    E. Add recombinant granulocyte–monocyte–colony-stimulating factor to his regimen

16. Which of the following is the proposed mechanism of renal calculi formation during chronic topiramate therapy?

    A. Increased gut absorption of calcium

    B. Inhibition of the enzyme carbonic anhydrase

    C. Renal calcium leak

    D. Increased absorption of oxalate from the colon

    E. Body fat and water loss

17. A 44-year-old man with bipolar disorder is transferring care to you. Before seeing you, he was receiving care at an indigent clinic. The patient is now able to afford psychiatric visits and medications because he got approved for Social Security disability. He is taking delayed release divalproex sodium 750 mg twice a day along with 40-mg citalopram and 2-mg lorazepam. The patient's clinical status is fairly stable; however, he asks whether he can take divalproex once a day instead of twice daily. You offer him the option of switching over to divalproex extended release formulation (divalproex-ER). Which of the following considerations must be borne in mind while switching the patient from delayed release divalproex to divalproex-ER?

    A. The patient will need a reduced dose of the extended release formulation dose to avoid toxicity

    B. Valproate (VPA) concentration from a blood sample drawn 12 to 15 hours after once-nightly administration of divalproex-ER is an accurate reflection of trough VPA concentrations

    C. The patient will need an increased dose of the extended release formulation to maintain therapeutic VPA levels

    D. Patients must be warned about a greater risk for sedation with the extended release formulation

    E. Increase in the risk of hepatotoxicity

18. A 46-year-old man with bipolar disorder along with chronic renal failure is recommended hemodialysis. The patient has a history of severe intolerance and/or nonresponse to alternative mood stabilizers. He is currently taking 900 mg of lithium per day in divided doses, which has significantly helped stabilize his mood swings and maintain his functioning. His nephrologist contacts you for recommendations regarding lithium therapy during hemodialysis. All of the following statements regarding lithium and hemodialysis are true EXCEPT:

    A. Maintenance doses of lithium are given three times weekly at the beginning of each dialysis session

    B. Lithium circulates unchanged in the body between dialysis sessions

    C. Lithium levels during dialysis are usually drawn 2 to 3 hours post dose

    D. Dialysis patients experience fluid shifts, and hence, monthly lithium levels are recommended

    E. None of the above

19. You see a 36-year-old man with treatment-resistant schizophrenia who is transferring care to the veteran health care system. He reports a 3-year-old history of treatment with brand name clozapine (Clozaril). He is taking 400 mg per day of the drug in divided doses. He is also on 10-mg zolpidem and 75-mg venlafaxine for his comorbid depressive symptoms. Overall, his symptoms appear to be stable and in partial remission. Other than sialorrhea, he denies any acute side effects to his medications. The Veterans Affair (VA) Pharmacy System prompts you to switch him over to generic clozapine. Which of the following statements should be the most important consideration when switching this patient from brand name clozapine to generic clozapine?

  A. Possible loss of therapeutic effect because of the presence of nonidentical active ingredient in the generic version

  B. Possibility of side effects because of the presence of nonidentical inactive ingredients in the generic version

  C. Possibility of lower bioequivalence because of the presence of nonidentical inactive ingredients in the generic version

  D. Cost savings in prescription drug costs associated with the generic version

  E. Increased frequency of hematologic monitoring is indicated following the conversion of brand name clozapine to generic clozapine

20. A 34-year-old man presents with major depressive features and psychotic symptoms. He has comorbid obsessive-compulsive symptoms. He is currently on 40-mg citalopram and 10-mg zolpidem. You decide to start him on 2 mg of risperidone. He has no personal or family history of diabetes or other metabolic problems. As per the American Diabetes Association (ADA)/American Psychiatric Association (APA) consensus management guidelines, what is the recommended monitoring schedule for fasting plasma glucose levels in this patient?

  A. Baseline, 4 weeks, 12 weeks, and annually

  B. Baseline, 8 weeks, 12 weeks, and annually

  C. Baseline, 12 weeks, and annually

  D. Baseline, 8 weeks, quarterly, and annually

  E. Baseline, quarterly, and annually

21. Which of the following is an active metabolite of venlafaxine?

    A. S-desmethylvenlafaxine

    B. O-desmethylvenlafaxine

    C. N-desmethylvenlafaxine

    D. N,O-didesmethylvenlafaxine

    E. C-desmethylvenlafaxine

22. Which of the following statements is not true regarding desvenlafaxine?

    A. No titration is required while starting the recommended dose

    B. Side effects occur in the first week of therapy

    C. Gastrointestinal (GI) side effects may be more frequent in women than in men

    D. Most common side effect is nausea

    E. Moderate interaction with the cytochrome P450 (CYP) system

23. All of the following statements regarding dystonia are true EXCEPT:

    A. It generally occurs within 4 to 7 days

    B. Old age is a major risk factor

    C. It is not seen with clozapine therapy

    D. Tardive dystonia responds well to clozapine

    E. Dystonia generally occurs after an increase in the neuroleptic dose

24. Buspirone acts on which of the following receptors?

    A. α_2-Adrenergic receptors

    B. Serotonin (5-HT$_1$A) receptors

    C. Dopamine D$_1$ receptors

    D. γ-Aminobutyric acid type A (GABA$_A$) receptors

    E. Muscarinic receptors

25. Which of the following is true regarding NMS?

  A. The risk for recurrence on reexposure to neuroleptic is approximately 30%

  B. Recurrence of NMS may be minimized by delaying rechallenge by 2 weeks post NMS

  C. A comorbid diagnosis of affective disorder is a risk factor for NMS

  D. Dehydration is a risk factor for NMS

  E. All of the above

26. Which of the following antidepressants has favorable effect on weight loss and little or no sexual side effect?

  A. Mirtazapine

  B. Fluoxetine

  C. Bupropion

  D. Nortriptyline

  E. Paroxetine

27. Which of the following plasma clozapine levels may be a useful guide to optimally efficacious dosage?

  A. Plasma levels >200 ng per ml

  B. Plasma levels >350 ng per ml

  C. Plasma levels >450 ng per ml

  D. Plasma levels >500 ng per ml

  E. Plasma levels >550 ng per ml

28. All of the following are side effects of carbamazapine EXCEPT:

    A. Benign pruritic rash

    B. Ataxia

    C. Hepatitis

    D. Nephrogenic diabetes insipidus

    E. Blurred vision

29. Which of the following is a not a dose-dependent side effect of VPA?

    A. Pancreatitis

    B. Nausea

    C. Weight gain

    D. Hand tremors

    E. Reversible elevations in liver enzymes

30. Which of the following statements is true regarding clozapine?

    A. Improve polydipsia and hyponatremia

    B. Improve negative symptoms

    C. Stabilize mood

    D. Reduce hostility and aggression

    E. All of the above

31. A 32-year-old man with panic disorder comes to you with severe anxiety attacks. He reports feeling anxious in crowded places such as malls and supermarkets. During his attacks, he would hyperventilate to the point where he would feel paresthesia and perioral tingling. He has been to several emergency rooms (ERs), and his medical evaluations have shown a slight subnormal calcium levels; however, no parathyroid or thyroid pathology was uncovered. You decide to prescribe him citalopram and lorazepam for his panic attacks. Lorazepam would act on central GABA receptor and exert its action through modulation of which of the following ion release?

  A. Sodium

  B. Calcium

  C. Potassium

  D. Chloride

  E. Magnesium

32. Which of the following anticholinergic agents has the least abuse potential?

  A. Trihexyphenidyl

  B. Benztropine

  C. Diphenhydramine

  D. Scopolamine

  E. Biperiden

33. All of the following are true regarding VPA therapy in a woman of childbearing age EXCEPT:

  A. All women without contraception should receive concomitant folate supplementation

  B. Folate should be administered throughout the gestation

  C. Vitamin K supplementation should be considered during the last month of gestation

  D. Serum concentration of VPA should not exceed 150 μg per ml

  E. None of the above

34. A 33-year-old man with major depression presents for treatment. In addition to other symptoms, he complains of initial and middle insomnia. You prescribe sertraline and temazepam for his condition. Which of the following scenarios is true regarding his condition and his treatment with temazepam?

    A. Depression is associated with increased REM density, although temazepam has no effect on REM sleep

    B. Depression and temazepam increase REM sleep

    C. Depression is associated with increased REM density, and temazepam suppresses REM sleep

    D. Depression and temazepam decrease REM sleep

    E. Depression and temazepam both have no effect on REM sleep

35. Which of the following drugs causes tolerance and withdrawal symptoms?

    A. Lorazepam

    B. Guanfacine

    C. Clonidine

    D. Phenobarbital

    E. All of the above

36. Which of the following is an α_2-adrenergic agonist?

    A. Yohimbine

    B. Clonidine

    C. Reserpine

    D. Mirtazapine

    E. All of the above

37. A 36-year-old man with bipolar disorder comes in with complaints of bilateral hand tremors and diarrhea. He is taking 1,200-mg lithium and 20-mg paroxetine (Paxil). He denies any recent change to his medications and/or alteration in his fluid intake, caffeine, or alcohol consumption. He has a history of rapid cycling bipolar disorder and is prone to quick relapses. The tremors have been quite bothersome, especially in social settings. What is the next best step in the management of this patient's bipolar disorder?

    A. Ask him to limit caffeine intake, and schedule him for a follow-up visit in 2 months

    B. Check his lithium level, and in a week, contact him with the results

    C. Reduce the dose of lithium to 1,000 mg and follow-up in 2 months

    D. Treat his tremors as worsening anxiety and increase paroxetine to 30 mg

    E. Prescribe him cyproheptadine to treat the diarrhea

38. All of the following are low potency conventional antipsychotic drugs EXCEPT:

    A. Thioridazine

    B. Chlorpromazine

    C. Trifluoperazine

    D. Mesoridazine

    E. Triflupromazine

39. All of the following are risk factors of tardive dyskinesia (TD) EXCEPT:

    A. Male sex

    B. Old age

    C. Affective disorder

    D. Diabetes mellitus

    E. Neuroleptic exposure for >6 months

40. A 45-year-old man with a diagnosis of schizophrenia along with treatment-resistant symptoms was recently started on clozapine. His symptoms improved considerably over a period of 2 months. At his 3-month follow-up visit, a complete blood cell count (CBC) reveals an ANC of 700 and WBC of 1,800. A decision to discontinue clozapine is made. You inform the patient that he may experience agitation, headache, nausea, or vomiting after the discontinuation of the drug. These symptoms are most likely to occur as a result of clozapine's action on which of the following receptors?

    A. Dopaminergic

    B. Muscarinic

    C. Serotonergic

    D. Adrenergic

    E. Histaminergic

41. Which of the following β-adrenergic receptor antagonists can be used as an augmenting agent in the treatment of depression?

    A. Propranolol

    B. Labetalol

    C. Pindolol

    D. Sotalol

    E. Nadolol

42. Mr. A, a 55-year-old white man, with major depression and new onset psychotic features is started on risperidone. He has been taking citalopram 40 mg for the past 4 months with partial symptom relief. His medical history is significant for closed-angle glaucoma and nocturnal polyuria. Within a week of taking risperidone, he develops perioral tremors. What is the most appropriate diagnosis of his tremor?

    A. Akinesia

    B. Rabbit syndrome

    C. TD

    D. Akathisia

    E. Drug-induced parkinsonism

43. Selective serotonin reuptake inhibitor (SSRI)-induced sexual side effects can be treated with which of the following drugs?

    A. Cyproheptadine

    B. Amantadine

    C. Buspirone

    D. Mianserin

    E. All the above

44. All of the following are complications of lithium therapy during the perinatal period EXCEPT:

    A. Cardiac arrhythmias

    B. Nephrogenic diabetes insipidus

    C. Oligohydramnios

    D. Floppy infant syndrome

    E. Thyroid function impairment

45. Which of the following is true regarding phenelzine?

    A. Plasma levels of phenelzine is under genetic control

    B. Slow acetylators appear to be more prone to side effects from phenelzine

    C. N-acetyltransferase appears to be inherited in a Mendelian fashion

    D. Ethnospecific loci of point mutations is responsible for slow acetylation

    E. All of the above

46. All of the following drugs can cause withdrawal syndrome EXCEPT:

    A. Propranolol

    B. Clonidine

    C. Fluoxetine

    D. Paroxetine

    E. Venlafaxine

47. All of the following can cause life-threatening anticholinergic intoxication syndrome when taken with benztropine EXCEPT:

    A. Dopamine receptor antagonists

    B. Tricyclics

    C. ß-Adrenergic receptor antagonists

    D. MAOIs

    E. Tetracyclics

48. Carbamazepine may decrease the drug plasma concentration of all of the following drugs, including carbamazepine itself, EXCEPT:

    A. Clozapine

    B. Lamotrigine

    C. Ethosuximide

    D. Fluoxetine

    E. Nefazodone

49. All of the following are clinical indications for the use of ß-adrenergic receptor antagonists EXCEPT:

    A. Lithium-induced postural tremor

    B. SSRI-induced anorgasmia

    C. Tricyclic-induced tremor

    D. Akathisia secondary to neuroleptics

    E. Aggressive behavior in schizophrenia and head injury

50. All of the following are true regarding clozapine EXCEPT:

    A. Strong D_1 and D_4 antagonism

    B. Weak D_2 antagonism

    C. 5-HT$_2$ antagonist

    D. D_2 receptor supersensitivity

    E. Highly anticholinergic

51. A 41-year-old white man is admitted in ICU for altered mental status. You are unable to interview the patient. On physical examination, he has increased bowel sounds. He has myoclonus, dilated pupils, and hyper-reflexia. Patient is on numerous medications, and his psychiatric medications include citalopram, risperidone, buspirone, and trazodone. His PCP recently started him on low-dose aspirin and tramadol. No other medical causes are identified. Which of the following drugs has a therapeutic role in the management of his condition?

    A. Cyproheptadine

    B. Benztropine

    C. Quetiapine

    D. Carbamazepine

    E. Bromocriptine

52. Which of following drugs can be used in the management of anxiety?

    A. Meprobamate

    B. Paraldehyde

    C. Glutethimide

    D. Butalbital

    E. Methohexital

53. Which of the following antihistamines can be used in the treatment of eating disorders?

    A. Promethazine

    B. Diphenhydramine

    C. Hydroxyzine

    D. Cyproheptadine

    E. Procyclidine

54. Flumazenil is useful in the reversal of all of the following medication overdoses EXCEPT:

    A. Zaleplon

    B. Zolpidem

    C. Lorazepam

    D. Phenobarbital

    E. Alprazolam

55. A 37-year-old white man with a history of major depression and panic disorder is currently taking alprazolam 1 mg twice a day and sertraline 20 mg every day. Patient complains of intolerable sexual side effects with sertraline. On reviewing his past history, it is noted that he developed seizures on bupropion and could not tolerate the sedation associated with mirtazapine. He was started on nefazodone. After 2 weeks of therapy with nefazodone, patient developed slurred speech, confusion, and ataxia. What is the most likely cause of these symptoms?

    A. Alprazolam toxicity

    B. Hepatic encephalopathy

    C. Serotonin syndrome

    D. Nefazodone toxicity

    E. None of the above

56. Mr. A, a 55-year-old white man, with major depression and new onset psychotic features is started on risperidone. He has been taking citalopram 40 mg for the past 4 months with partial symptom relief. His medical history is significant for closed-angle glaucoma and nocturnal polyuria. Within a week of taking risperidone, he develops perioral tremors. What is the most appropriate treatment for Mr. A's new onset movement disorder?

    A. Trihexyphenidyl

    B. Benztropine

    C. Amantadine

    D. Procyclidine

    E. Diphenhydramine

57. Benzodiazepine and nonbenzodiazepine hypnotic drugs bind to the $GABA_A$ receptor and exert their action by which of the following mechanism?

    A. Triggering the influx of chloride into the cell and thus creating an inhibitory effect on neuronal cells

    B. Increasing the affinity of GABA for its receptor site and thus enhancing the channel opening effect

    C. Triggering the influx of potassium into the neuronal cell and thus causing the cell membrane to be hyperpolarized

    D. Create a conformational change in the GABA receptor such that both GABA and dopamine act as agonists

    E. Triggering the influx of sodium into the neuronal cell and thus causing the cell membrane to be hyperpolarized

58. All of the following statements are true regarding lithium therapy during pregnancy EXCEPT:

   A. Risk of Ebstein anomaly after prenatal lithium exposure rises from 1 in 20,000 to 1 in 1,000

   B. In women with mild and infrequent episodes of illness, lithium therapy should be gradually (>2 weeks) tapered before conception

   C. In women with severe episodes but at moderate risk for relapse in the short term, lithium therapy should be tapered before conception but reinstituted after 7 to 9 weeks

   D. Lithium should be restarted in the second trimester in women with severe episodes and at moderate risk of relapse

   E. Women with severe and frequent episodes of illness, lithium should be continued throughout gestation in conjunction with counseling regarding reproductive risks

59. A 32-year-old African American man with treatment-resistant schizophrenia is being considered for clozapine therapy. His current medications are risperidone, clonazepam, lithium, quetiapine, and benztropine. Which of the following medications when given with clozapine has the potential to increase the risk of asterixis?

   A. Clonazepam

   B. Benztropine

   C. Risperidone

   D. Lithium

   E. Quetiapine

60. Ramelton acts on melatonin receptors—MT_1 and MT_2—that are located in which area of the brain?

   A. Suprachiasmatic nucleus

   B. Ventral tegmental area

   C. Basal ganglia

   D. Amygdala

   E. Hippocampal area

61. Which of the following antihistamines acts both on histamine and serotonin receptors?

    A. Promethazine

    B. Diphenhydramine

    C. Hydroxyzine

    D. Cyproheptadine

    E. Benztropine

62. What is the best choice for treating insomnia in breast-feeding women?

    A. Ativan

    B. Zolpidem

    C. Zaleplon

    D. Temazepam

    E. None of the above

63. All of the following statements are true regarding sodium oxybate (Xyrem) EXCEPT:

    A. It is indicated in the treatment of excessive daytime sleepiness

    B. Used for cataplexy in patients with narcolepsy

    C. It is taken at bedtime and again 2.5 to 4 hours later

    D. Food significantly enhances the bioavailability of sodium oxybate

    E. It is a schedule III drug under the Controlled Substances Act

64. To reduce the neonatal risks, it is recommended that the dose of VPA should not exceed more than

    A. 500 mg per day

    B. 800 mg per day

    C. 1,200 mg per day

    D. 1,400 mg per day

    E. 1,600 mg per day

65. All of the following statements regarding lamotrigine-induced Steven–Johnson syndrome are true EXCEPT:

    A. The incidence in adults is about 0.1%

    B. The risk is higher with concomitant phenytoin therapy

    C. The risk is higher if the dosage is escalated too rapidly

    D. Most cases appear after 2 to 8 weeks of therapy

    E. Rarely it may be associated with multiple organ failure

66. Which of the following statements is true regarding carbamazepine-induced hyponatremia?

    A. It is a likely result of carbamazepine's antidiuretic effect

    B. It is common in children

    C. It occurs in 1% of patients taking carbamazepine

    D. It is common in male gender

    E. All of the above

67. Which of the following drugs' absorption is enhanced when taken with food?

    A. Diazepam

    B. Carbamazepine

    C. Ziprasidone

    D. Vilazodone

    E. All of the above

68. Which of the following mood stabilizers should be avoided as a first-line agent in women of childbearing age?

    A. Lithium

    B. VPA

    C. Carbamazepine

    D. Lamotrigine

    E. Oxcarbazepine

69. Electrocardiographic (ECG) changes occur with which of the following antipsychotic drugs' therapy?

    A. Thioridazine

    B. Pimozide

    C. Chlorpromazine

    D. Ziprasidone

    E. All of the above

70. Which of the following medications should be avoided in a patient taking clozapine?

    A. Captopril

    B. Carbamazepine

    C. Sulfonamides

    D. Propylthiouracil

    E. All of the above

71. Which of the following statements is not true regarding antipsychotic drugs?

    A. Conventional antipsychotic agents increase c-fos in nucleus accumbens and striatum

    B. Atypical agents increase c-fos in prefrontal cortex

    C. Conventional agents block 75% to 90% of D_2 receptors, whereas clozapine blocks only 40% to 60%

    D. Atypical agents produce depolarization blockade both in A_9 and A_{10} dopamine neurons

    E. The A_{10} mesolimbic pathway is possibly associated with psychosis

72. Lithium can mitigate which of the following adverse effects of carbamazepine?

    A. Syndrome of inappropriate antidiuretic hormone

    B. Leukopenia

    C. CNS toxicity

    D. Bone marrow suppression

    E. Rash

73. Which of the following percentages most closely resembles the incidence of SSRI-resistant obsessive-compulsive disorder (OCD)?

    A. 5%

    B. 10%

    C. 40%

    D. 60%

    E. 80%

74. Which of the following is the most likely mechanism of neutropenia associated with carbamazepine therapy?

    A. Inhibition of colony-stimulating factor in the bone marrow

    B. Fibrosis of the bone marrow

    C. Idiosyncratic reaction

    D. Autoimmune destruction of the bone marrow

    E. Marginalization and sequestration

75. Which of the following statements is not true regarding nonbenzodiazepine hypnotic drugs?

    A. Zaleplon has a rapid onset of action and short duration

    B. Zaleplon has a half-life of >6 hours

    C. Zaleplon is absorbed slowly when taken after fatty meal

    D. Zolpidem is a selective $GABA_A$ receptor α_1-subunit agonist

    E. Risk of dependence with zolpidem increases with the duration of treatment

76. Which of the following statements is true regarding eszopiclone?

    A. It is structurally related to zaleplon

    B. It is the R (–) enantiomer of zopiclone

    C. It is safe in pregnancy

    D. Unpleasant taste is a very common side effect

    E. All of the above

77. Which of the following sets of side effects is possible as a result of a drug–drug interaction (DDI) between tramadol and paroxetine?

    A. Hypotension, decreased tendon reflexes, and arrhythmias

    B. Seizures, hyperthermia, and enhanced analgesic effect of tramadol

    C. Mental status changes, hypertension, and myoclonus

    D. Arrhythmia and cardiac arrest

    E. Respiratory arrest

78. Lithium was reported to be effective in mania by

    A. Lowell Randall

    B. Leo Sternbach

    C. John Cade

    D. Arvid Carlsson

    E. Emil Kraepelin

79. A 27-year-old African American woman is brought in by the squad after an overdose with amitriptyline. ECG shows dysrhythmia. Besides supportive measures, adding which of the following is recommended first-line agent in the management of dysrhythmia induced by TCA overdose?

   A. Ammonium chloride

   B. Lidocaine

   C. Sodium bicarbonate

   D. Physostigmine

   E. All of the above

80. Which of the following actions of tricyclics is/are responsible for its toxicity during overdose?

   A. Antagonism at adrenergic receptors

   B. Norepinephrine reuptake inhibition

   C. Membrane-stabilizing effect on the myocardium

   D. Antagonism at cholinergic receptors

   E. All of the above

81. Pharmacokinetics, one of the principles that determines the clinical efficacy of a drug, is described as

   A. Genetic differences in the behavioral response to pharmacologic agents

   B. What the drug does to the body

   C. What the body does to the drug

   D. Genetic differences in the absorption and degradation of drugs

   E. Genetic differences in tissue sensitivity to drugs

82. In addition to declining WBC and ANC counts, which of the following is an indication for interrupting clozapine therapy?

    A. Monocytosis

    B. Eosinophilia

    C. Thrombocytopenia

    D. Polycythemia

    E. All of the above

83. Which of the following is a known complication of chronic SSRI use?

    A. Subjective sense of fatigue

    B. Yawning

    C. Exhaustion

    D. Concentration problems

    E. All of the above

84. A 44-year-old man with schizoaffective disorder is prescribed clozapine for his treatment-resistant symptoms. He is also on zolpidem for insomnia. His medical history is significant for obesity. He was hospitalized for pneumonia. During this hospitalization, he was started on fluvoxamine for depressed mood. You see him in your clinic 2 weeks after discharge. As an astute clinician, you recognize the potential for an important DDI between clozapine and fluvoxamine. You decide to see him more frequently and even order a clozapine serum level. The DDI between clozapine and fluvoxamine involves which of the following cytochrome enzymes?

    A. CYP2D6

    B. CYP2C9

    C. CYP3A4

    D. CYP1A2

    E. CYP2C19

85. Which of the following neurotransmitters is postulated to mediate changes in weight associated with psychotropic drugs?

    A. Histamine

    B. Serotonin

    C. Dopamine

    D. Norepinephrine

    E. All of the above

86. All of the following are risk factors for seizure during bupropion therapy EXCEPT:

    A. History of head trauma

    B. History of seizure disorder

    C. History of liver cirrhosis

    D. History of febrile seizures during childhood

    E. History of eating disorder

87. A 36-year-old man with schizophrenia is currently stable on aripiprazole. The patient visited his PCP 2 weeks ago for weight loss, night sweats, fatigue, and chronic cough. He tested positive for purified protein derivative (PPD), and the chest X-ray was suggestive of pulmonary tuberculosis. After confirmation of the diagnosis, he was started on isonicotinylhydrazine (INH) and rifampicin. Today he appears more detached, suspicious, and aloof. He also appears to be reacting to internal stimuli. You suspect a drug interaction. Which of the following is the next best action?

    A. Stop aripiprazole and start him on a different antipsychotic

    B. Increase the dose of aripiprazole

    C. Increase the dose of rifampicin

    D. Start clozapine

    E. None of the above

88. All of the following drugs are associated with hyponatremia EXCEPT:

    A. Oxcarbazepine

    B. Citalopram

    C. Carbamazepine

    D. Lamotrigine

    E. Amitriptyline

89. Which of the following drugs has high therapeutic index?

    A. Lithium

    B. Haloperidol

    C. Nortriptyline

    D. Carbamazepine

    E. All of the above

90. All of the following are true regarding psychotropics and dialysis EXCEPT:

    A. Hemodialysis is the best treatment for VPA overdose

    B. Hemodialysis is indicated in overdose with venlafaxine

    C. Drugs with low protein binding are good candidates for dialysis

    D. Drugs with high protein binding are not cleared during dialysis

    E. Mainstay treatment of lithium toxicity is hemodialysis

91. All of the following are risk factors for torsades de pointes during paren-
teral administration of haloperidol therapy EXCEPT:

    A. Hyperkalemia

    B. Hypomagnesemia

    C. Liver failure

    D. Congestive heart failure (CHF)

    E. Hypoxia

92. A 45-year-old woman with major depression and chronic pain is on
amitriptyline, citalopram, and zolpidem. She continues to experience depressive symptoms despite being on 60-mg citalopram for 12 weeks. Her
psychiatrist decides to discontinue citalopram and starts her on a second
antidepressant. After 2 weeks on the new drug, she develops urinary
retention and her ECG shows conduction abnormalities. The second
antidepressant is most likely to be which of the following?

    A. Bupropion

    B. Mirtazapine

    C. Sertraline

    D. Fluvoxamine

    E. None of the above

93. All of the following are advantages of guanfacine over clonidine
EXCEPT:

    A. Less sedating

    B. Less frequent dosing

    C. Less severe withdrawal/discontinuation symptoms

    D. Availability of transdermal preparation

    E. None of the above

94. What is the prevalence of Ebstein anomaly during lithium therapy in first trimester?

    A. 1% to 2%

    B. 0.05% to 0.1%

    C. <0.5%

    D. 2% to 5%

    E. 5% to 8%

95. What is the half-life of immediate-release venlafaxine?

    A. 8 hours

    B. 4 hours

    C. 3 hours

    D. 6 hours

    E. 12 hours

96. Which of the following TCAs is devoid of sedative effects?

    A. Nortriptyline

    B. Protriptyline

    C. Desipramine

    D. Doxepin

    E. None of the above

97. All of the following statements regarding duloxetine are true EXCEPT:

  A. The drug can affect urethral resistance

  B. The drug is potent inhibitor of neuronal serotonin and norepinephrine reuptake

  C. It is indicated in the treatment of fibromyalgia

  D. The drug is mainly metabolized by the CYP3A4 P450 isozyme

  E. None of the above

98. Which of the following statements regarding selegiline transdermal patch is true?

  A. Orthostatic hypotension is the most common side effect with the drug

  B. The drug is Food and Drug Administration (FDA) approved for bipolar depression

  C. No dietary restrictions are required when dosed at 6 mg per 24 hours

  D. When used in children, dietary modifications are required at any dose

  E. All of the above

99. A 34-year-old woman comes to your office with symptoms suggestive of OCD. There are no comorbid psychotic symptoms. You decide to prescribe drug X based on its robust efficacy and safety in treating OCD. As the patient is about to leave your office, she states, "Doc, I forgot to mention, I suffered a head injury about 2 years ago and have experienced brief periods of amnesia and twitching of my eyelids." This new information prompts you to reconsider prescribing drug X. Which of the following agents is most likely to be drug X?

  A. Aripiprazole

  B. Clomipramine

  C. Mirtazapine

  D. Bupropion

  E. Clozapine

100. Which of the following drugs has the greatest evidence for causing depression as an unwanted side effect?

    A. Isotretinoin

    B. Oral contraceptives

    C. Atenolol

    D. Varenicline

    E. Digoxin

101. Which of the following TCAs has a greater inhibitory effect on norepinephrine reuptake compared with serotonin reuptake?

    A. Doxepin

    B. Nortriptyline

    C. Imipramine

    D. Amitriptyline

    E. Clomipramine

102. A 43-year-old woman on tamoxifen therapy develops symptoms of depression. Which of the following antidepressants is best indicated in her treatment?

    A. Bupropion

    B. Paroxetine

    C. Venlafaxine

    D. Fluoxetine

    E. Duloxetine

103. Which of the following statements regarding management of bipolar depression is/are true?

   A. Results from the Systematic Treatment Enhancement Program for Bipolar Disorder (STEP-BD) study showed higher rates of treatment-emergent affective switches with mood stabilizer + adjunctive antidepressant versus mood stabilizer + placebo

   B. Results from the STEP-BD study showed the statistical difference in outcome by adding antidepressants to mood stabilizer when compared with mood stabilizers and placebo

   C. STEP-BD data suggest that addition of intensive psychotherapy (cognitive behavior therapy, interpersonal therapy, and family-focused therapy) to standard mood stabilizer treatment was no better than mood stabilizer treatment without these treatments

   D. Quetiapine is FDA approved for the treatment of acute bipolar depression

   E. All of the above

104. You see a 50-year-old patient with schizophrenia in community mental health setting. His caseworker is very concerned about his poor medication compliant. The patient has had frequent outpatient visits and periodic symptom exacerbation. None of them have resulted in inpatient hospitalization though. The patient is currently prescribed 10 mg of haloperidol daily and 100 mg of divalproex sodium. You do not see any evidence of TD or other extrapyramidal symptoms. The patient agrees to a trial of injectable haloperidol decanoate. Which of the following is the most appropriate starting dose of haloperidol decanoate?

   A. 100 mg

   B. 50 mg

   C. 300 mg

   D. 200 mg

   E. 250 mg

105. Which of the following high-potency benzodiazepines is known to have long half-life?

    A. Diazepam

    B. Chlordiazepoxide

    C. Clonazepam

    D. Lorazepam

    E. Temazepam

106. Risperidone's therapeutic efficacy is related to its antagonism of dopamine type 2 and serotonin type 2 receptors. The drug's side effect of orthostatic hypotension is related to its binding affinity for which of the following receptor sites?

    A. H_1 histaminergic receptors

    B. M_1 muscarinic receptors

    C. α-Adrenergic receptors

    D. β-Adrenergic receptors

    E. Serotonin 5-HT_3 receptors

107. Bupropion is clinically useful in all of the following conditions EXCEPT:

    A. Major depressive disorder

    B. Tobacco cessation

    C. Opiate dependence

    D. Attention deficit hyperactivity disorder

    E. SSRI-induced sexual dysfunction

108. Which of the following medications has demonstrated efficacy in the management of acute mania?

    A. Lamotrigine

    B. Gabapentin

    C. Carbamazepine ER (Equetro)

    D. Clonazepam

    E. All of the above

109. All of the following statements regarding treatment adherence during antidepressant therapy is true EXCEPT:

    A. Most patients discontinue antidepressants after consulting with their physician

    B. Most studies have found that 20% to 50% of patients discontinue antidepressant medication within the first few months of therapy

    C. Patients with comorbid posttraumatic stress disorder (PTSD) and anxiety disorders are less likely to adhere to antidepressant medications

    D. Tolerability issues during antidepressant treatment are one of the main reasons for nonadherence

    E. Complicated dosing schedule negatively influences antidepressant adherence

110. Which of the following analgesics can be safely used in a patient on selegiline transdermal patch?

    A. Tramadol

    B. Morphine

    C. Propoxyphene

    D. Codeine

    E. All of the above

111. Which of the following antidepressants has an ascending dose-antidepressant response curve?

    A. Nefazodone

    B. Sertraline

    C. Paroxetine

    D. Mirtazapine

    E. Bupropion

112. All of the following can be used in the treatment of neuroleptic-induced akathisia EXCEPT:

    A. Benzodiazepines

    B. Propranolol

    C. Clonidine

    D. Prochlorperazine

    E. Benztropine

113. Which of the following statements is true regarding thyroid augmentation in unipolar depression?

    A. Serum levels of free T_3 can clearly predict preferential response to thyroid augmentation

    B. The dose for T_3 for thyroid augmentation is typically 25 to 50 μg per day

    C. The evidence base for T_3 augmentation of TCAs and SSRIs is equal and comparable

    D. T_3 augmentation is safe in the presence of cardiac disease

    E. An adequate trial of T_3 augment is at least 4 to 6 weeks

114. All of the following drugs could increase lithium levels when administered together EXCEPT:

    A. Verapamil

    B. Ramipril

    C. Hydrochlorothiazide

    D. Naproxen

    E. Theophylline

115. You are called to evaluate a 54-year-old white woman with a history of bipolar disorder for altered mental status and bizarre behavior. The patient is acutely confused, lethargic, and near mute; she begins to urinate on the floor and attempts to remove her prosthetic eye. The patient is currently taking divalproex-ER 1,000 mg at bedtime. On review of her records, you note that she was recently started on topiramate for prophylaxis of her migraine headaches. Her serum VPA level is 80 mg per dl, her serum ammonia is 80 μmol per L, and her transaminases are normal. There is no history of any recent CNS pathology, dietary changes, or preexisting metabolic issues that could potentially explain her symptoms. Which of the following is the most likely explanation for her symptoms?

    A. As a result of a DDI

    B. Acute nutritional deficiency

    C. Development of new onset psychiatric symptoms

    D. Acute hepatic failure

    E. All of the above

116. You manage the care of a 44-year-old woman with schizophrenia who is currently taking 4 mg risperidone once daily for her symptoms. She has been on risperidone for the past 2 years with good symptom control. She reports to you that her breasts appear engorged and that at times she can express milk from them. You ask her if she could be pregnant, to which she replies, "Doc, you don't have to worry about that as I attained menopause about a year ago." She also jokes on how she does not have to worry about using contraception anymore. You order a prolactin level test, thyroid function test, and check her urine for pregnancy. Her prolactin level comes back as 140 ng per ml, whereas the rest of her lab workup is normal. After weighing pros and cons and patient preferences, you decide to start her on aripiprazole and cross tapering risperidone. After 4 weeks of aripiprazole therapy, her prolactin level comes back as 15 ng per ml. You should particularly warn the patient of which of the following in the ensuing few months.

    A. Risk of worsening psychosis

    B. Risk of pregnancy

    C. Risk of blurred vision

    D. Nausea

    E. Risk of low bone mineral density

117. All of the following statements regarding osmotic-controlled release oral delivery system (OROS) drug delivery technology are true EXCEPT:

    A. OROS technology allows for reduced peak and trough fluctuations

    B. OROS enables the use of an effective starting dose without the need for dose titration

    C. OROS technology does not facilitate reduced dosing frequency

    D. Long-acting oral paliperidone and methylphenidate formulations utilize OROS technology

    E. Drugs delivered by OROS technology have lower potential for drug abuse

118. Which of the following phases of the pharmacokinetic sequence is affected by pregnancy?

 A. Absorption

 B. Distribution

 C. Metabolism

 D. Excretion

 E. All of the above

119. Which of the following antidepressants when administered during pregnancy has a statistically higher odds ratio for cardiovascular malformations?

 A. Fluoxetine

 B. Paroxetine

 C. Citalopram

 D. Sertraline

 E. Bupropion

120. All of the following medications act as serotonin (5-HT) and norepinephrine reuptake inhibitors EXCEPT:

 A. Duloxetine

 B. Milnacipran

 C. Venlafaxine

 D. Mirtazapine

 E. Amitriptyline

121. Which of the following drugs has the greatest risk of QTc prolongation?

    A. Risperidone

    B. Quetiapine

    C. Ziprasidone

    D. Olanzapine

    E. Aripiprazole

122. Which of the following MAOIs tends to be activating/stimulating?

    A. Tranylcypromine

    B. Phenelzine

    C. Selegiline

    D. Maprotiline

    E. Linezolid

123. What percentage of patients enrolled in the Clinical Antipsychotic Trials of Intervention Effectiveness (CATIE) had metabolic syndrome as defined by the National Cholesterol Education Program?

    A. 25%

    B. 41%

    C. 60%

    D. 15%

    E. 5%

124. Which of the following medications has little or no evidence in the treatment of fibromyalgia?

    A. Milnacipran

    B. Duloxetine

    C. Cyclobenzaprine

    D. Nonsteroidal anti-inflammatory drugs (NSAIDs)

    E. Pregabalin

125. Which of the following conclusions from the Sequenced Treatment Alternatives to Relieve Depression (STAR*D) study is most accurate?

    A. Patients who received cognitive-behavioral therapy (CBT) as either a switch or augmentation had lower response rates compared with pharmacotherapy

    B. A majority of the patients achieved remission with antidepressant monotherapy within 4 weeks

    C. The probability of relapse during continuation therapy increased as a function of the number of treatment trials required to achieve remission

    D. Patients who do not respond to an SSRI have greater probability of responding to an antidepressant with a different mechanism of action versus another SSRI

    E. All of the above

126. All of the following laboratory screening tests are recommended before initiating carbamazepine for the treatment of bipolar disorder EXCEPT:

    A. CBC

    B. Hepatic function tests

    C. Renal functions tests

    D. ECG

    E. TSH

127. At what minimum dose does trazodone inhibit the serotonin transporter (SERT) and act as a potent antidepressant in addition to a hypnotic?

    A. 100 mg

    B. 250 mg

    C. 150 mg

    D. 300 mg

    E. 600 mg

128. The hematologic change most frequently associated with lithium therapy is

    A. Leukopenia

    B. Leukocytosis

    C. Agranulocytosis

    D. Aplastic anemia

    E. Thrombocytopenia

129. You are the treating psychiatrist for a 38-year-old male surgeon with OCD. The patient is currently on 60-mg citalopram, which he is tolerating fairly well. He developed intolerable side effects to prior trials of venlafaxine and bupropion. The patient finds his symptoms distressing and at times quite disabling. You recommend augmentation with the atypical antipsychotic risperidone. The patient mentions the AmpliChip CYP450 test for genotyping CYP isoenzymes genes. You reluctantly agree that the test could aid your treatment strategy. The patient's test results show inactivation of both alleles of the CYP2D6 gene. On the basis of this information, which of the following treatment approaches would make sense?

    A. Prescribe risperidone at approximately half the usual starting dose

    B. Prescribe risperidone at approximately one-half times the usual starting dose

    C. Lower the dose of citalopram while starting him on the usual adult starting dose of risperidone

    D. Decide not to use risperidone in this case

    E. Discard the information as not standard clinical care and do nothing

130. Which of the following statements is/are true regarding the use of prazosin in the treatment of PTSD?

    A. Prazosin is the most lipid soluble of the α_1-blockers

    B. Prazosin has shown to decrease recurrent distressing as well as to improve sleep quality in PTSD

    C. Prazosin is associated with the first-dose phenomenon

    D. Prazosin can increase the risk of priapism when concurrently administered with trazodone

    E. All of the above

131. As per the ADA/APA consensus guidelines, all of the following are recommended metabolic monitoring guidelines for patients either starting or changing atypical antipsychotics EXCEPT:

    A. Monitor body mass index (BMI) at baseline, 4, 8, and 12 weeks and quarterly thereafter

    B. Monitor fasting blood glucose at baseline, 12 weeks, and annually

    C. Monitor fasting lipid profile at baseline, 12 weeks, and annually

    D. Monitor BP at baseline, 12 weeks, and annually

    E. Monitor TSH at baseline and annually

132. Which of the following medications carries a black box warning for suicidal thinking and behavior (suicidality) in adults?

    A. Risperidone

    B. Ziprasidone

    C. Aripiprazole

    D. Olanzapine

    E. All of the above

133. A 36-year-old Caucasian man with schizophrenia discontinues all his medications and insists that his 18-year-old son needs to be castrated. He believes that male members of his family are possessed by demons and is afraid that his son might pass it on to the next generation. His wife is extremely concerned and requests immediate treatment. You gather a history of failed trials of aripiprazole and quetiapine. You decide to start risperidone and titrate him to 2 mg twice a day over a 3-week period. There are no indications for hospitalization. After a week, his wife calls requesting you to consider olanzapine because her sister-in-law is doing well on it. What should be your next best step?

    A. Increase the dose of risperidone to 3 mg twice a day

    B. Stop risperidone and start olanzapine

    C. Continue the same dose of risperidone

    D. Taper risperidone as you start olanzapine 5 mg at bedtime

    E. Refer for electroconvulsive therapy (ECT)

134. Which of the following benzodiazepines has the shortest half-life?

A. Flurazepam

B. Triazolam

C. Temazepam

D. Clonazepam

E. Diazepam

135. Atypical antipsychotics increase the risk of which of the following?

A. Type 2 diabetes mellitus

B. Weight gain

C. Risk of strokes in elderly patients

D. Hyperlipidemia

E. All of the above

136. A 43-year-old African American man with a diagnosis of generalized anxiety disorder (GAD) and seizure disorder is on chronic therapy with alprazolam and carbamazepine. He is pretty tolerant of the medication regimen and reports doing well. Carbamazepine is discontinued after blood cell counts suggests aplastic anemia and divalproex is started. Over the next couple of weeks, he develops ataxia, slurred speech, and confusion. Which of the following is the most likely cause for the emergence of this set of symptoms?

A. Alprazolam toxicity

B. Carbamazepine discontinuation syndrome

C. Disseminated intravascular coagulation secondary to divalproex-induced thrombocytopenia

D. Complex partial seizures

E. Transient ischemic attack (TIA)

137. Which of the following antipsychotic medications has the highest selectivity and potency for dopamine D_2 receptors?

    A. Quetiapine

    B. Pimozide

    C. Loxapine

    D. Thioridazine

    E. Ziprasidone

138. The potential cause of sleepwalking as a side effect of zolpidem is because of which of the following effects?

    A. Increased REM sleep

    B. Decreased REM sleep

    C. Increased slow-wave sleep

    D. Decreased slow-wave sleep

    E. Increased REM latency

139. Which of the following statements regarding topiramate is true?

    A. Topiramate is a carbonic anhydrase inhibitor

    B. Topiramate can cause metabolic alkalosis as a side effect

    C. Topiramate is efficacious in bipolar mania

    D. Topiramate increases intestinal absorption of calcium and thus causing renal stones

    E. Topiramate is not efficacious in prophylaxis of migraine headaches

140. You see a 40-year-old man with bipolar disorder who is currently taking lithium carbonate 900 mg at bedtime. His most recent serum level is 0.7 mEq per L. He is tolerating the medication fairly well and reports adequate symptoms control. He recently saw his PCP who diagnosed him with hypertension and started on him a diuretic. Among the following diuretic agents, which one can affect lithium levels the most?

    A. Furosemide

    B. Mannitol

    C. Hydrochlorothiazide

    D. Spironolactone

    E. Atenolol

141. Symptoms arising from which of the following organ systems is a key differentiating factor between the hypertensive reaction and histamine headache, both of which can occur with an MAOI?

    A. GI system

    B. Ocular

    C. Vascular system

    D. CNS

    E. Endocrine system

142. Weight gain, a side effect with mirtazapine therapy, is mediated through the blockade of which of the following receptors?

    A. $5\text{-HT}_2\text{A}$

    B. $5\text{-HT}_2\text{C}$ and H_1 histaminergic

    C. 5-HT_3

    D. M_1 muscarinic

    E. All of the above

143. A 38-year-old white man with a long history of restless legs associated with painful sensations in the legs seeks a neurologist's opinion. He feels that his PCP does not take his complaints seriously. His symptoms are worse at night and while at rest. He is a school bus driver, and he has at times experienced cramping in his legs while driving and has had to pull off the road. He is very worried that he might get into a motor vehicle accident (MVA), especially with children on board. He also complains of daytime tiredness, mood disturbance, and inability to perform daily activities such as travelling long distances, and he is frustrated that he cannot go to movies any longer. He is diagnosed with restless legs syndrome and started on pramipexole. He comes in a few days later, reporting that he developed an irresistible sleep attack that occurred suddenly, and he barely avoided a major MVA. He is flustered and anxious and worried that he might lose his job. Which of the following is the best explanation for his symptoms?

    A. Narcolepsy

    B. Drug-induced sleep attack

    C. Conversion disorder

    D. Panic attack

    E. Excessive daytime sedation with pramipexole

144. Buspirone is more advantageous compared with benzodiazepines in which of the following clinical aspects?

    A. Convenience of once a day dosing

    B. Provides rapid relief from anxiety symptoms

    C. Has low risk for abuse

    D. Can be used to augment antipsychotics drugs

    E. All of the above

145. Which of the following statements regarding TCAs are/is true?

    A. Amitriptyline has maximal anticholinergic property among the tricyclics

    B. Desipramine has the least anticholinergic property among the tricyclics

    C. Doxepin has potent H_1 antagonistic properties

    D. Nortriptyline has a curvilinear therapeutic window

    E. All of the above

146. All of the following are risk factors for NMS EXCEPT:

    A. Dehydration

    B. Agitation

    C. Low serum iron

    D. Potency of neuroleptic

    E. None of the above

147. Which of the following is the best-studied medications till date for borderline personality disorder (BPD)?

    A. Fluoxetine

    B. Divalproex sodium

    C. Aripiprazole

    D. Lamotrigine

    E. Quetiapine

148. Which of the following antidepressants has the most evidence for safety during breast-feeding?

A. Citalopram

B. Venlafaxine

C. Bupropion

D. Nortriptyline

E. Paroxetine

149. Which of the following antidepressants has significant secondary benefits as an antipruritic agent?

A. Doxepin

B. Mirtazapine

C. Nortriptyline

D. Paroxetine

E. Desipramine

150. Which of the following is the best established nonpsychiatric use of lithium?

A. Treatment of cluster headaches

B. Reducing chemotherapy-associated neutropenia

C. Reducing hematopoietic toxicity associated with zidovudine use

D. Treatment of herpes simplex infections

E. Treatment of the syndrome of inappropriate secretion of antidiuretic hormone (SIADH)

151. Which of the following animal models is being used as an antidepressant screening tests?

    A. The learned helplessness model

    B. Reward model

    C. Behavioral despair/forced swim paradigm

    D. Genetic models

    E. All of the above

152. Which of the following is the side effect of mirtazapine?

    A. Somnolence

    B. Increase in serum cholesterol

    C. Rare incidence of neutropenia

    D. Weight gain

    E. All of the above

153. Carbamazepine therapy may be associated with all of the following EXCEPT:

    A. Decrease in T_3 and T_4

    B. Decrease in serum cholesterol

    C. Impaired dexamethasone suppression test

    D. False positive pregnancy tests

    E. Risk of skin rash

154. The nonbenzodiazepine drug zolpidem exerts its action by binding to which of following GABA$_A$ receptor units?

    A. α1-Subunit

    B. β1-Subunit

    C. γ2S-Subunit

    D. η-Subunit

    E. None of the above

155. SSRI-induced sexual side effects can be managed with which of the following medications?

    A. Aripiprazole

    B. Venlafaxine

    C. Bupropion

    D. Mirtazapine

    E. All the above

156. Which of the following is an additive risk factor for the development of renal calculi during topiramate therapy?

    A. Coadministration of acetazolamide

    B. Coadministration of furosemide

    C. Coadministration of lithium

    D. Coadministration of divalproex

    E. All of the above

157. Which of the following antipsychotic agents may have a role in the development and progression of cataract?

   A. Risperidone

   B. Olanzapine

   C. Quetiapine

   D. Aripiprazole

   E. Haloperidol

158. Which of the following is used to treat TCA-induced peripheral anticholinergic signs and symptoms?

   A. Methacholine

   B. Carbachol

   C. Bethanechol

   D. Benztropine

   E. Diphenhydramine

159. Which of the following antidepressants is most likely to cause increased sweating as a side effect?

   A. Bupropion

   B. Mirtazapine

   C. Venlafaxine

   D. Nefazodone

   E. All of the above

160. Which of the following medications has a role in the management of antidepressant-induced sweating?

    A. Benztropine

    B. Propranolol

    C. Guanfacine

    D. Lorazepam

    E. All of the above

161. All of the following are antipsychotics belonging to the phenothiazine class EXCEPT:

    A. Trifluoperazine

    B. Chlorpromazine

    C. Thiothixene

    D. Mesoridazine

    E. Fluphenazine

162. A 29-year-old man with schizophrenia is currently stable on a combination of aripiprazole and divalproex sodium. He attends a day program and has been very compliant with his treatment. His past medical history is remarkable for a recent bout of upper respiratory infection for which he is prescribed clarithromycin. You see him after he has been taking the antibiotic for 4 days; he appears more anxious and reports worsening tremors and blurred vision. You suspect a drug interaction involving aripiprazole and erythromycin. The putative DDI involves which of the following cytochrome enzyme?

    A. CYP2D6

    B. CYP2C9

    C. CYP3A4

    D. CYP2C19

    E. CYP4D

163. Which of the following hematologic abnormalities is seen during clozapine therapy?

    A. Macrocytosis

    B. Thrombocytopenia

    C. Anemia

    D. Polycythemia

    E. Granulocytopenia

164. Rechallenge of clozapine is not permitted with which of the following counts?

    A. ANC reaches 2,000 per mm

    B. ANC reaches 1,000 per mm

    C. ANC reaches 1,500 per mm

    D. WBC count reaches 2,000 per mm

    E. WBC count reaches 2,500 per mm

165. Which of the following drugs inhibits the CYP2D6 isoenzyme?

    A. Bupropion

    B. Fluvoxamine

    C. Risperidone

    D. Desipramine

    E. Desvenlafaxine

166. Which of the following drugs strongly inhibits the CYP2D6 isoenzyme?

    A. Bupropion

    B. Fluvoxamine

    C. Risperidone

    D. Desipramine

    E. Fluoxetine

167. Which of the following cytochrome enzymes is more abundant in the gut wall as well as in the liver?

    A. CYP3A4

    B. CYP2D6

    C. CYP2C9

    D. CYP2C19

    E. CYP2E1

168. P-glycoprotein transport plays an important role in determining blood concentrations and bioavailability of psychotropic drugs. Which of the following statements regarding p-glycoprotein is true?

    A. Inhibition of p-glycoprotein within the gut wall results in increased drug efficacy

    B. Inhibition of p-glycoprotein within the gut wall results in decreased drug efficiency

    C. Induction of p-glycoprotein within the gut wall results in increased drug efficacy

    D. P-glycoprotein is exclusively located in the plasma membrane of gut lumen

    E. None of the above

169. Which of the following drugs antagonizes 5-TH$_1$A receptors?

    A. Mirtazapine

    B. Ziprasidone

    C. Buspirone

    D. Vilazodone

    E. Asenapine

170. Which of the following benzodiazepines is not safe in hepatic insufficiency?

   A. Oxazepam

   B. Lorazepam

   C. Temazepam

   D. Flurazepam

   E. None of above

171. All of the following are true regarding lithium EXCEPT:

   A. Comorbid substance abuse is a predictor of poor response to lithium

   B. Lithium is not well tolerated in the elderly population

   C. Lithium is not as effective as anticonvulsants in the treatment of rapid cycling bipolar disorder

   D. Lithium is as effective as antipsychotics in bipolar disorder with comorbid psychotic symptoms

   E. Lithium therapy is not recommended in patients with a history of poor compliance

172. A 39-year-old Caucasian man with schizophrenia is on clozapine therapy for the past 2 years. He failed several medication trials for anxiety and continues to experience anxiety and irritability. You decide to prescribe buspirone for his symptoms. Three weeks following buspirone therapy, he started complaining of nausea and epigastric pain. All of the following are the potential side effects resulting from the combination of clozapine and buspirone EXCEPT:

   A. Thrombocytopenia

   B. Hyperglycemia

   C. GI tract bleeding

   D. Anemia

   E. None of the above

173. Which of the following psychotropic medications may lead to kidney stones formation?

    A. Topiramate

    B. Depakote

    C. Lamotrigine

    D. Oxcarbazepine

    E. All of the above

174. First-pass effect refers to which of the following aspects of a medication's metabolism?

    A. Redistribution

    B. Lipid solubility

    C. Elimination half-life

    D. Presystemic elimination

    E. Rate of intestinal absorption

175. The risk of teratogenic neural tube defects is greatest for the offspring of mothers taking which of the following anticonvulsants?

    A. Phenytoin

    B. Lamotrigine

    C. VPA

    D. Levetiracetam

    E. Carbamazepine

176. A 42-year-old Caucasian man is admitted to the emergency department following an overdose of lithium carbonate. He is semiresponsive and complains of nausea and abdominal discomfort. His physical examination shows hyperreflexia and ECG T-wave flattening. He has history of CHF as well. The serum lithium level is 2.6 mEq per L. Which of the following is the most appropriate treatment?

    A. Sodium bicarbonate IV

    B. Hemodialysis

    C. 0.9% Sodium chloride IV

    D. Mannitol IV

    E. Gastric lavage

177. The most common side effect during MAO therapy is

    A. Sexual dysfunction

    B. Excessive flatus

    C. Postural hypotension

    D. Peripheral edema

    E. Asthenia

178. Clozapine is associated with which of the following cardiovascular effects?

    A. QTc prolongation

    B. Myocarditis

    C. Cardiomyopathy

    D. Pericarditis

    E. All of the above

179. Among the following drugs used in mood disorder, which has been most strongly associated with cognitive side effects?

    A. Lamotrigine

    B. Olanzapine

    C. Topiramate

    D. Carbamazepine

    E. VPA

180. Weight gain is not a problem with which of the following antipsychotics?

    A. Olanzapine

    B. Risperidone

    C. Quetiapine

    D. Molindone

    E. Chlorpromazine

181. All of the following statements regarding clozapine are true EXCEPT:

    A. Patients are eligible for monthly WBC monitoring after 12 months of continuous therapy with clozapine without any abnormal hematologic counts

    B. The CBC results may not be >7 days old for pharmacist to dispense clozapine

    C. Clozapine is schedule II drug

    D. In the event that a patient discontinues clozapine, weekly blood work for 4 weeks (minimum) must be performed

    E. Clozapine has an FDA warning for increased risk of death in elderly patients with dementia-related psychosis

182. What is the maximum recommended daily dose of intramuscular (IM) ziprasidone?

    A. 60 mg per day

    B. 40 mg per day

    C. 160 mg per day

    D. 100 mg per day

    E. 160 mg per day

183. Peak plasma concentrations of IM olanzapine are typically reached in

    A. 45 to 60 minutes

    B. 15 to 30 minutes

    C. 60 to 90 minutes

    D. <15 minutes

    E. None of the above

184. All of the following are criteria for treatment-refractory schizophrenia proposed by Kane et al. EXCEPT:

    A. No episodes of good functioning in the previous 5 years

    B. Total Brief Psychiatric Rating Scale (BPRS) score of >45

    C. Failure to respond to at least three antipsychotic trials from two different chemical class of adequate duration and dose

    D. Failure to tolerate to a trial of haloperidol

    E. Failure to respond to a trial of long-acting injectable antipsychotic agent

185. What dose of fluoxetine has shown to be effective in reducing binge eating and purging in bulimic women?

    A. 10 mg per day

    B. 20 mg per day

    C. 40 mg per day

    D. 60 mg per day

    E. 120 mg per day

186. You manage care of a 34-year-old woman with bipolar type II disorder and recently start her on lamotrigine. The patient reports doing well on 150 mg lamotrigine per day with no side effects. She forgets to refill her prescription on trip to Mexico and calls to report being off her medication for 12 days. Which of the following statements is true regarding restarting lamotrigine following interruption of therapy?

    A. In case of interruption of lamotrigine therapy for 7 days, it requires prior initial start-up dose and gradual retitration

    B. In case of interruption of lamotrigine therapy for 2 weeks, it requires prior initial start-up dose and gradual retitration

    C. In case of interruption of lamotrigine therapy for >4 weeks, it requires prior initial start-up dose and gradual retitration

    D. In case of interruption of lamotrigine therapy, restart to prior initial start-up dose and gradual onset is necessary only when there is a skin rash

    E. None of the above

187. Which of the following is rare but recognized side effect of clozapine?

    A. Dilated cardiomyopathy

    B. Myocarditis

    C. Heart failure

    D. Sudden cardiac death

    E. All of the above

188. You manage a 31-year-old woman with a history of major depression and BPD with multiple impulsive suicide attempts by drug overdose. She has been to the ER several times for her parasuicide behavior. She has been poorly compliant with your attempts to engage her in a dialectical behavior therapy (DBT) program. Knowing that the availability of the drug is an important factor motivating the choice of the drug used for intentional drug overdose, you should take all the following precautions EXCEPT:

    A. Issue prescriptions of short duration

    B. Prescribe multiple but low doses of psychotropic medications

    C. Evaluate the appropriateness of prescribing psychotropic medications in this particular case

    D. Avoid prescribing TCA

    E. None of the above

189. Which of the following antidepressants has the most seizurogenic potential?

    A. Bupropion

    B. Paroxetine

    C. Venlafaxine

    D. Mirtazapine

    E. All of the above

190. What is the effect of food on the bioavailability of ziprasidone?

    A. Increase in bioavailability

    B. Minimize gastric disease

    C. Decrease in bioavailability

    D. No change in bioavailability of ziprasidone

    E. None of the above

191. All of the following drugs have been reported to decrease WBC counts EXCEPT:

    A. Olanzapine

    B. Mirtazapine

    C. Clozapine

    D. Carbamazepine

    E. None of the above

192. All of the following are true regarding modafinil EXCEPT:

    A. Modafinil has reinforcing properties at higher dose

    B. Modafinil is a racemic compound, whose enantiomers have different pharmacokinetics

    C. Modafinil is listed in schedule IV of the Controlled Substances Act

    D. Headache is a common side effect of modafinil

    E. Modafinil is indicated for narcolepsy

193. Which of the following statements is true regarding venlafaxine and BP elevation?

    A. The incidence of sustained hypertension with venlafaxine is dose dependent

    B. The incidence of sustained hypertension with venlafaxine is not dose dependent

    C. The incidence of sustained hypertension is higher with extended release than immediate-release preparation

    D. The BP elevation is transient and will resolve with chronic therapy

    E. All of the above

194. Which of the following drugs acts as a $GABA_B$ receptor agonist?

    A. Diazepam

    B. Zolpidem

    C. Eszopiclone

    D. Baclofen

    E. All of the above

195. Which of the following drugs has the greater evidence for upregulating neurotrophins including brain-derived neurotrophic factor (BDNF), nerve growth factor, and neurotrophin-3 (NT3), supporting its usefulness as a robust neuroprotective agent?

    A. Clozapine

    B. Lithium

    C. Memantine

    D. Vitamin E

    E. *Ginkgo biloba*

196. Prodopaminergic agents may have a useful role in the treatment of anergic depression. Furthermore, there is growing evidence that mood disorders may be associated with neuronal plasticity and cellular resilience. Which of the following agents by virtue of its prodopaminergic and neurotrophic effects has shown promise in the treatment of bipolar disorder and unipolar depression?

    A. Bupropion

    B. Pramipexole

    C. Lithium

    D. Aripiprazole

    E. Clozapine

197. Depression occurs in approximately 50% of patients with Parkinson disease. Which of the following antidepressants has the greatest evidence in the treatment of this condition?

   A. Nortriptyline

   B. Bupropion

   C. Pramipexole

   D. Sertraline

   E. Venlafaxine

198. Which of the following psychiatric drugs has demonstrated efficacy in the treatment of acute and delayed chemotherapy-induced nausea and vomiting in patients receiving emetogenic chemotherapy?

   A. Doxepin

   B. Venlafaxine

   C. Fluoxetine

   D. Olanzapine

   E. Aripiprazole

199. All of the following are true regarding selegiline EXCEPT:

   A. Used for Parkinson disease and depression

   B. It is an MAO-B inhibitor that becomes MAO-A inhibitor at higher doses

   C. SSRIs are contraindicated

   D. Weight loss is reported with selegiline therapy

   E. None of the above

200. A 36-year-old African American male was diagnosed with major depressive disorder with atypical features and was started on phenelzine with significant benefit. His symptoms responded well to phenelzine, and his functioning improved. Which of the following should be avoided to prevent hypertensive crisis?

  A. Amphetamine

  B. Methyldopa

  C. Methylphenidate

  D. Buspirone

  E. All of the above

201. Which of the following antidepressants is associated with a rare but dangerous side effect of severe hepatotoxicity, sometimes requiring liver transplant?

  A. Nefazodone

  B. Desvenlafaxine

  C. Desipramine

  D. Paroxetine

  E. Tranylcypromine

202. Which of the following drugs has data suggesting efficacy in the treatment of menopausal hot flashes?

  A. Venlafaxine

  B. Desipramine

  C. Bupropion

  D. Prazosin

  E. Clonazepam

203. Which of the following is true regarding lithium-induced hypothyroidism?

  A. It is associated with high prevalence of thyroid autoantibodies

  B. Lithium is known to suppress thyroid functions in about 10% of patients

  C. Prevalence of clinical hypothyroidism is higher in men when compared with women

  D. Elevated TSH level during lithium treatment is an indication for discontinuing lithium

  E. All of the above

204. A patient whose hypertension is well controlled on clonidine presents with major depression. Which of the following antidepressants should be avoided in the treatment of his depression?

  A. Fluoxetine

  B. Paroxetine

  C. Nortriptyline

  D. Bupropion

  E. None of the above

205. In 2005, the FDA approved the first pharmacogenetic test using DNA array technology for genotyping CYP isoenzymes genes. The AmpliChip CYP450 test (Roche Molecular Systems) genotypes which of the following isoenzymes?

  A. CYP2D6 and CYP2C19

  B. CYP2D6 and CYP3A4

  C. CYP2D6 and CYP1A2

  D. CYP2D6, CY2C19, CYP34A, and CYP1A2

  E. All of the above

206. Which of the following is true regarding effects of lithium therapy on renal function?

- **A.** Lithium irreversibly reduces kidneys' urine-concentrating ability
- **B.** The renal effects are unrelated to the dose of lithium
- **C.** Lithium-induced polyuria is rare among patients treated with lithium
- **D.** Lithium inhibits vasopressin-stimulated cyclic AMP (cAMP) production, which is one of the primary factors contributing to the impaired urine-concentrating ability
- **E.** All of the above

207. Dantrolene has a role in the management of which of the following conditions?

- **A.** NMS
- **B.** Serotonin syndrome
- **C.** Catatonia
- **D.** Heat stroke
- **E.** Metabolic myopathy

208. Combined VPA and carbamazepine therapy may pose which of the following risk factors?

- **A.** VPA increases the concentration of 10 to 11 epoxide metabolites of carbamazepine
- **B.** VPA clearance is increased, and hence, increased VPA dose may be required
- **C.** Toxicity may emerge even at therapeutic serum carbamazepine (CBZ) levels
- **D.** Symptoms such as ataxia, nystagmus, and headache may emerge
- **E.** All of the above

209. Which of the following psychotropic drugs has the best evidence for decreasing the suicide risk in schizophrenia?

    A. Lithium

    B. Clozapine

    C. Aripiprazole

    D. Fluoxetine

    E. Olanzapine

210. All of the following are true regarding VPA-induced hepatotoxicity EXCEPT:

    A. Children younger than 2 years are most vulnerable

    B. Hepatotoxicity usually occurs during the first 6 months of treatment

    C. Carnitine supplementation may prevent the onset of hepatotoxicity

    D. VPA-induced hepatic dysfunction resolves completely after discontinuing the drug

    E. None of the above

211. Which of the following drugs has a wide therapeutic index?

    A. Alprazolam

    B. Amitriptyline

    C. Lithium

    D. Clozapine

    E. Carbamazepine

212. Which of the following antipsychotic drugs can cause pigmentary retinopathy?

    A. Chlorpromazine

    B. Thioridazine

    C. Quetiapine

    D. Molindone

    E. Olanzapine

213. Treatment with which of the following antipsychotics has shown to have either a very rapid (<6 weeks) or a delayed (6 weeks to 6 months) clinical response?

    A. Aripiprazole

    B. Clozapine

    C. Paliperidone

    D. Molindone

    E. Haloperidol

214. Which of the following psychotropic drugs has the best evidence for decreasing the suicide risk in bipolar disorder?

    A. Clozapine

    B. Aripiprazole

    C. Lithium

    D. Fluoxetine

    E. All of the above

215. Desipramine is the main metabolite of which of the following?

    A. Clomipramine

    B. Imipramine

    C. Nortriptyline

    D. Amitriptyline

    E. None of above

216. Which of the following is a dopamine receptor agonist?

    A. Pergolide

    B. Ropinirole

    C. Bromocriptine

    D. Pramipexole

    E. All of the above

217. Which of the following antidepressants has little to no evidence in treating neuropathic pain?

    A. Amitriptyline

    B. Venlafaxine

    C. Paroxetine

    D. Duloxetine

    E. Nortriptyline

218. Which of the following medications is FDA approved for the treatment of irritability associated with autistic disorder?

    A. Olanzapine

    B. Risperidone

    C. Quetiapine

    D. Ziprasidone

    E. Asenapine

219. Which of the following statements regarding dosing guidelines for long-acting risperidone depot preparation is/are true?

    A. Dose adjustments can be made every 2 weeks

    B. Oral supplementation with oral antipsychotic must continue for the first week of therapy

    C. The maximum dose should not exceed 50 mg every 2 weeks

    D. Clinical effect from a dosage adjustment can be expected within a week following the injection of the higher dose

    E. All of the above

220. Which of the following TCAs possesses the most serotonergic activity?

    A. Maprotiline

    B. Clomipramine

    C. Nortriptyline

    D. Desipramine

    E. Protriptyline

221. Which of the following drugs is contraindicated in patients with a history of allergy to TCAs?

    A. Carbamazepine

    B. Lamotrigine

    C. Trifluoperazine

    D. Mirtazapine

    E. Topiramate

222. All of the following statements regarding neuroleptic-induced TD are true EXCEPT:

   A. Anticholinergic medications can decrease TD movements

   B. Clonazepam has shown to be useful in TD

   C. Clozapine can decrease TD movements

   D. Botulinum toxin is not a general treatment for TD

   E. Recognition of TD should be followed by immediate discontinuation of the antipsychotic medication

223. All of the following are true regarding aripiprazole EXCEPT:

   A. It is a dopamine–serotonin system stabilizer

   B. Partial agonist at D_2

   C. Full agonist at 5-HT_2A

   D. Partial agonist at 5-HT_1A

   E. None of the above

224. A 39-year-old Caucasian man is admitted to medical department with suspected nosocomial pneumonia caused by *Staphylococcus aureus*. The primary team consults you for the management of his worsening anxiety and nightmares. You interview the patient and find out that he has been diagnosed with combat-related PTSD and is currently taking a combination of clonidine, trazodone, and ziprasidone for his symptoms. You also note the infectious disease consultation recommending treatment with the antibiotic linezolid. Which of the following statements regarding his management is most accurate?

   A. Prescribe sertraline because it is FDA-approved drug for PTSD

   B. Discontinue trazodone because it may precipitate symptoms of hypertension, hyperthermia, and mental status changes

   C. Discontinue clonidine because it may precipitate symptoms of hypotension, thrombocytopenia, and bradycardia

   D. Discontinue ziprasidone because it may precipitate symptoms of mental status changes, myoclonus, and diarrhea

   E. None of the above

225. Which of the following statements is true regarding fluvoxamine?

    A. Minimal inhibitory effect of CYP1A2 isoenzyme

    B. The drug is eliminated from systemic circulation primarily by renal excretion as unchanged drug

    C. Binds less extensively to plasma proteins

    D. Fluvoxamine is an FDA category B drug to be used in pregnancy

    E. All of the above

226. Which of the following is the most appropriate treatment for clozapine-induced hypersalivation?

    A. Dose reduction

    B. Chewing gum

    C. Anticholinergic agents

    D. α_2-Agonist

    E. All of the above

227. Which of the following benzodiazepines is highly lipophilic?

    A. Chlordiazepoxide

    B. Diazepam

    C. Lorazepam

    D. Temazepam

    E. Alprazolam

228. As per the ADA/APA consensus management guidelines, what is the recommended monitoring schedule for BMI for patients receiving atypical antipsychotics?

    A. Baseline, 12 weeks, and annually

    B. Baseline, 4 weeks, 8 weeks, 12 weeks, and quarterly

    C. Baseline, 4 weeks, 8 weeks, 12 weeks, and annually

    D. Baseline, 8 weeks, quarterly, and annually

    E. Baseline, quarterly, and annually

229. All of the following clinical strategies is/are helpful in reducing the incidence of antipsychotic-induced TD EXCEPT:

    A. Using lowest effective dose of antipsychotic

    B. Prophylactic anticholinergic medications

    C. Abnormal Involuntary Movement Scale (AIMS) exam every 6 months

    D. Switch to clozapine if TD appears

    E. Supplement with vitamin 800 IU per day

230. Which of the following characteristics is suggestive of a benign skin eruption during therapy with lamotrigine?

    A. Maculopapular rash

    B. Facial and neck involvement

    C. Purpuric appearance

    D. Tender rash

    E. Internal organ involvement

231. All of the following are potential adverse effects during VPA therapy EXCEPT:

    A. Hair loss

    B. Polycystic ovary disease

    C. Pancreatitis

    D. Thrombocytopenia

    E. None of the above

232. All of the following regarding lamotrigine are true EXCEPT:

    A. Lamotrigine primarily inhibits sodium channels

    B. Pregnancy increases lamotrigine clearance

    C. The greatest risk of rash with lamotrigine is during the first 2 weeks of treatment

    D. The drug's bioavailability is not altered by food

    E. Lamotrigine may cause hematologic adverse reactions such as thrombocytopenia

233. All of the following are true regarding CYP isoenzymes EXCEPT:

    A. They are located on microsomal membranes

    B. They oxidatively metabolize prostaglandins and fatty acids

    C. They oxidatively metabolize medications

    D. They are found predominantly in gut and brain

    E. They metabolize all psychotropic medications except lithium

234. Which of the following TCAs inhibits norepinephrine reuptake the most?

    A. Desipramine

    B. Protriptyline

    C. Nortriptyline

    D. Doxepin

    E. Clomipramine

235. The most common renal side effect during lithium therapy is

    A. Enuresis

    B. Polyuria

    C. Urgency

    D. Hematuria

    E. Oliguria

236. A 38-year-old Caucasian woman with a history of major depressive disorder without psychotic features is well maintained on fluoxetine (Prozac) 40 mg per day. Her past medical history is significant for long QTc syndrome. She was rear-ended in a motor vehicle accident and sustained a whiplash injury. Which of the following should be used with caution in treating her current condition?

    A. Acetaminophen

    B. Baclofen

    C. Cyclobenzaprine

    D. Ibuprofen

    E. Oxycodone

237. Electroencephalogram of a patient on benzodiazepine is likely to show all of the following EXCEPT:

   A. Decrease in the REM sleep

   B. Decrease in stage III and IV sleep

   C. Shortened REM latency

   D. Increased K spindles in stage II

   E. None of the above

238. A 32-year-old Caucasian man with no earlier psychiatric diagnosis is brought to your clinic by his wife for depressed mood in the past 3 months. He graduated last year from an orthopedics residency program and joined a leading hospital in the town about 7 months ago. During the interview, the patient stated that he is living his dream now and questions whether there is anything more in terms of productive achievement. He stopped playing golf, which used to be his passion. He reports that he has no interest in life. He sleeps about 15 hours a day and complains that he has no energy left. At work, he could not concentrate and complains of decreased motor activity. His appetite has increased over the past 3 months. There is no significant past medical history, and he is currently not taking any medications. You diagnose him with major depressive episode and decide to start him on an antidepressant. Which of the following would be your preferred choice?

   A. Fluoxetine

   B. Sertraline

   C. Duloxetine

   D. Phenelzine

   E. Citalopram

239. All of the following statements regarding chloral hydrate are true EXCEPT:

    A. It is useful for initial insomnia

    B. It has no risk for addiction

    C. GI distress is a common side effect

    D. It may prolong prothrombin time in anticoagulated patients

    E. It is used as an analgesic

240. VPA may be a better choice over other mood stabilizers in bipolar patients presenting with which of the following?

    A. Mixed episodes

    B. Rapid cycling

    C. Comorbid substance abuse

    D. Impulsivity

    E. All of the above

241. The following are disadvantages of short half-life benzodiazepines EXCEPT:

    A. Rebound insomnia

    B. Anterograde amnesia

    C. Can be used in the treatment of benzodiazepine withdrawal syndrome

    D. Withdrawal symptoms on abrupt discontinuation

    E. Rebound anxiety

242. Which of the following drugs can produce withdrawal dyskinetic movements on sudden discontinuation after chronic therapy?

    A. Lithium

    B. Metoclopramide

    C. Cimetidine

    D. Bromocriptine

    E. Alprazolam

243. Which of the following statements is false regarding creatinine phosphokinase (CPK) elevations associated with NMS?

    A. Significant CPK elevations can occur with IM injections, physical restraints, and agitation

    B. Mild to moderate CPK elevation is not specific for NMS

    C. CPK elevation >1,000 IU per L is more specific for NMS

    D. Absence of CPK elevations rules out a diagnosis of NMS

    E. CPK elevation in NMS may vary between 1,000 and as high as 100,000 IU per L

244. Which of the following is contraindicated in patients on selegiline transdermal patch?

    A. Carbamazepine

    B. Oxcarbazepine

    C. Dextroamphetamine

    D. Methylphenidate

    E. All of the above

245. Cyclobenzaprine should be avoided with all of the following medications EXCEPT:

    A. Duloxetine

    B. Phenelzine

    C. Sertraline

    D. Fluoxetine

    E. None of the above

246. Postinjection delirium sedation syndrome (PDSS) is associated with which of the following depot antipsychotics?

    A. Risperidone depot preparation

    B. Olanzapine extended release injectable suspension

    C. Paliperidone palmitate

    D. Haloperidol decanoate

    E. Zuclopenthixol acetate

247. Which of the following agents used in the treatment of nightmares associated with PTSD is most notorious for producing a first-dose phenomenon?

    A. Trazodone

    B. Prazosin

    C. Olanzapine

    D. Cyproheptadine

    E. Zolpidem

248. A 35-year-old man presents with treatment refractory depression. He has failed treatments with paroxetine, citalopram, bupropion, and lithium augmentation. He refuses ECT treatments. On reviewing his medical chart, you note that his hypertension is being treated with clonidine. Which of the following treatments would be indicated in his case?

    A. Nortriptyline

    B. Venlafaxine

    C. Mirtazapine

    D. Repetitive transcranial magnetic stimulation (rTMS)

    E. Fluoxetine

249. All of the following regarding St. John's wort (SJW) are true EXCEPT:

    A. The presumed active component of SJW is hypericin

    B. SJW is a potent inhibitor of CYP3A4

    C. Transplant patients should not receive SJW

    D. SJW is better than placebo for the treatment of depression

    E. Concurrent use of SSRI and SJW may result in an increased risk of serotonin syndrome

250. Which of the following antidepressants would be a good choice for a depressed patient with significant nausea?

    A. Bupropion

    B. Citalopram

    C. Nortriptyline

    D. Mirtazapine

    E. Sertraline

251. All of the following statements regarding lithium-induced tremors are true EXCEPT:

    A. Lithium tremors respond to treatment with metoprolol

    B. Lithium tremors tend to be slow and rhythmic

    C. Lithium tremors present at rest

    D. Lithium tremors are made worse by movement

    E. None of the above

252. Which of the following benzodiazepines has the longest half-life?

    A. Temazepam

    B. Flurazepam

    C. Triazolam

    D. Diazepam

    E. Nitrazepam

253. Which of the following is the primary reason for monitoring plasma nortriptyline concentrations during the treatment of major depression?

    A. The existence of a curvilinear therapeutic window

    B. To monitor the risk of cardiac toxicity

    C. To monitor medication compliance

    D. Clinical correlation of efficacy and adequate dosing

    E. All of the above

254. According to positron emission tomography (PET) studies, what percentage of D_2 receptor occupancy correlates with maximal antipsychotic efficacy?

    A. 50% to 55%

    B. 20% to 30%

    C. 65% to 70%

    D. 40% to 50%

    E. 100%

255. Which of the following statements regarding the management of over-dose with TCAs is true?

    A. Dialysis is the first line of treatment

    B. Activated charcoal is helpful

    C. Prophylactic antiarrhythmics are indicated

    D. Ammonium chloride is the first line of treatment

    E. Lidocaine is the first line of treatment

256. Which of the following accurately describes lithium exposure and neonatal outcome?

    A. Stopping lithium 1 to 2 days before the delivery is likely to improve the neonatal outcomes

    B. Higher neonatal lithium levels are associated with significantly lower Apgar scores

    C. Higher neonatal lithium concentrations are associated with higher rates of CNS complications

    D. Higher neonatal lithium concentrations are associated with higher rates of neuromuscular complications

    E. All of the above

257. All of the following are sexual side effects seen in women receiving trazodone EXCEPT:

    A. Priapism of the clitoris

    B. Spontaneous orgasm

    C. Increased libido

    D. Decreased libido

    E. None of the above

258. Which of the following antipsychotic medications has the lowest propensity to lower the seizure threshold?

A. Haloperidol

B. Chlorpromazine

C. Molindone

D. Clozapine

E. None of the above

259. What is the estimated mortality rate with NMS?

A. <5%

B. 20% to 30%

C. 50% to 60%

D. 5% to 10%

E. 10% to 20%

260. All of the following are true regarding asenapine EXCEPT:

A. Neutral metabolic effects

B. Minimal effects on prolactin

C. Well tolerated

D. Lower extrapyramidal side effects

E. None of the above

261. All of the following statements are true regarding therapeutic drug monitoring with lithium EXCEPT:

   A. Steady state lithium levels are attained after 2 days of constant dosing

   B. Serum lithium levels 12 hours post dose are 30% higher in patients taking the sustained release (SR) preparation compared with the immediate release (IR) preparation

   C. There is a point of care/office-based test for serum lithium commercially available

   D. Therapeutic levels for the treatment of acute mania are in the range of 1.0 to 1.5 mEq per L

   E. It is not uncommon to see fluctuating serum lithium levels in geriatric patients in the absence of any dose changes in lithium

262. A 28-year-old Caucasian woman with bipolar disorder has been taking lithium 900 mg per day for the past 18 months. She has had two hospitalizations in the past 2 years but none after initiating lithium. She has failed several mood stabilizers including VPA, carbamazepine, and lamotrigine. She presents to the ER with nausea and vomiting. Physical examination is unremarkable. Lithium level is 1.1. Urine human chorionic gonadotropin is positive. Ultrasonography/ultrasonogram (USG) abdomen confirms 5-week-old gestational sac. Patient sounds very happy, but her boyfriend insists on terminating the pregnancy because of his concern of fetal malformations. After discussing the benefits and risks, they decide to continue with the pregnancy. All of the following preventative measures are recommended during pregnancy on lithium therapy EXCEPT:

   A. Fetal echocardiogram is recommended between 16 and 18 weeks of gestation

   B. Caution should be exercised regarding maternal NSAID

   C. NSAID should be avoided in neonates

   D. Withhold lithium therapy for 24 to 48 hours before delivery

   E. None of the above

263. Which of the following features is/are associated with PDSS?

    A. General malaise

    B. Ataxia

    C. Dysarthria

    D. Disorientation

    E. All of the above

264. Under which of the following conditions would ziprasidone be life threatening?

    A. QTc >500 milliseconds

    B. Heart failure

    C. Arrhythmias

    D. Recent myocardial infarction (MI)

    E. All of the above

265. Which of the following statements is true regarding leukopenia associated with carbamazapine therapy?

    A. It predisposes patients to infections

    B. It is a strong indicator of the development of agranulocytosis

    C. Incidence of leukopenia associated with carbamazapine therapy is 35%

    D. It resolves spontaneously despite continued treatment

    E. All of the above

266. Which of the following is the most common side effect with MAOI therapy?

    A. Hypertensive crisis

    B. Hypotension

    C. Weight gain

    D. Hypersomnia

    E. Tyramine reaction

267. All of the following drugs have been linked to serious exfoliative dermatitis, an adverse dermatologic effect, EXCEPT:

    A. Carbamazepine

    B. Lamotrigine

    C. Phenobarbital

    D. VPA

    E. None of the above

268. All of the following statements regarding the epileptogenic effects of bupropion are true EXCEPT:

    A. Most seizures with bupropion occur within the first several hours after taking the dose

    B. The drug's active metabolite threohydrobupropion is primarily responsible for the occurrence of seizures

    C. Exceeding 150 mg in any single dose is a risk factor for seizures

    D. History of closed head injury increases the risk of developing seizure

    E. None of the above

269. A 38-year-old man with schizophrenia on olanzapine and clonazepam therapy develops blasphemous obsessions and ritualized praying and counting. You diagnose him with comorbid OCD. Assuming you leave his current medications unchanged, which of the following drugs should be avoided in the treatment of his OCD?

    A. Fluoxetine

    B. Buspirone

    C. Fluvoxamine

    D. Paroxetine

    E. None of the above

270. All of the following are high-potency benzodiazepine EXCEPT:

    A. Alprazolam

    B. Clonazepam

    C. Temazepam

    D. Triazolam

    E. Lorazepam

271. Which of the following over-the-counter medications/food should not be used or used with caution in patients on selegiline transdermal patch?

    A. SJW

    B. Caffeine

    C. Chocolate

    D. Tobacco

    E. All of the above

272. Which of the following clinical observations is a result of mirtazapine's preferential blocking of the histamine-1 receptor at low doses, whereas at higher doses the drug blocks the α_2-adrenergic receptor?

    A. Weight gain on low-dose mirtazapine therapy versus weight loss on high-dose mirtazapine therapy

    B. Pronounced sedation on low-dose mirtazapine therapy rather than on high-dose mirtazapine therapy

    C. Low incidence of sexual side effects on low-dose mirtazapine therapy rather than on high-dose mirtazapine therapy

    D. Low incidence of triglyceridemia on low-dose mirtazapine therapy rather than on high-dose mirtazapine therapy

    E. All of the above

273. Coadministration of lithium and carbamazapine can cause the following additive side effects on all the following organ systems EXCEPT:

    A. CNS

    B. Endocrine

    C. Hematopoietic system

    D. Renal system

    E. None of the above

274. Which of the following is the assumed mechanism for antipsychotic-induced QTc prolongation and the risk of torsades de pointes?

    A. Blockade of the human ether-a-go-go-related gene (HERG) potassium channel

    B. Blockade of the HERG calcium channel

    C. Combined calcium and potassium channel blockade

    D. Combined sodium and potassium channel blockade

    E. All of the above

275. All of the following statements are true regarding the mechanism of action of lithium EXCEPT:

    A. Lithium causes a relative depletion of myoinositol in the brain

    B. Lithium significantly inhibits cAMP accumulation through G proteins

    C. Lithium alters fos expression through a protein kinase C (PKC) mechanism

    D. Lithium alters sodium transport in nervous system

    E. None of the above

276. A 32-year-old man with treatment-resistant schizophrenia was admitted to nonsmoking psychiatric ICU. After titrating him on clozapine, he was transferred to a step-down unit for another week. Two weeks after his discharge to his home, he relapsed and presented to the ER again. The DDI between clozapine and smoking involves which of the following cytochrome enzymes?

    A. CYP2D6

    B. CYP2C9

    C. CYP3A4

    D. CYP1A2

    E. CYP2C19

277. Management of akathisia includes all of the following EXCEPT:

    A. Propranolol

    B. Lowering the neuroleptic dose

    C. Clonazepam

    D. Diphenhydramine

    E. None of the above

278. A 34-year-old woman with bipolar disorder maintaining well on lithium carbonate comes to you with concerns about worsening acne. The patient reports trying several remedies for her acne; however, none of them have been successful. She appears very frustrated and makes mention of discontinuing lithium. Despite your reassurances, the patient insists on discontinuing lithium and requests you to prescribe an alternative mood stabilizer. You decide to start her on divalproex sodium. As the patient leaves your office, she makes mention of her recent visit to her PCP where she signed up for a program requiring her to commit to using two methods of contraception and having pregnancy tests each month. In return, she would get a medication for her severe acne. Which of the following concerns should be addressed before the patient leaves your office?

    A. Potential for reduced efficacy of her acne medication secondary to drug interactions with divalproex sodium

    B. Increased risk for depression and suicide from her acne medication

    C. Potential for a lithium discontinuation syndrome

    D. Potential for her acne medication to induce manic symptoms

    E. All of the above

279. Trazodone's most potent binding property is at which of the following sites?

    A. Serotonin 5-HT$_2$A receptor

    B. H$_1$ histamine receptor

    C. Serotonin 5-HT$_1$A receptor

    D. SERT

    E. All of the above

280. Which of the following statements is/are true regarding advantages of paliperidone palmitate depot antipsychotic over other available second-generation depot antipsychotics?

  A. Paliperidone palmitate is administered monthly

  B. Paliperidone palmitate does not require supplementation with oral antipsychotics

  C. Paliperidone palmitate does not require an additional precautionary observation period during the postinjection period

  D. Paliperidone palmitate prefilled syringes require no reconstitution or refrigeration

  E. All of the above

281. Drug interactions have known to occur between divalproex sodium and all of the following EXCEPT:

  A. Carbamazepine

  B. Lamotrigine

  C. Risperidone

  D. Aspirin

  E. Aripiprazole

282. Which of the following is an appropriate loading dose for sodium VPA in the management of acute mania?

  A. 15 mg/kg/day

  B. 20 mg/kg/day

  C. 50 mg/kg/day

  D. 35 mg/kg/day

  E. 40 mg/kg/day

283. Propranolol should not be combined with all of the following drugs EXCEPT:

   A. Thioridazine

   B. Haloperidol

   C. Levothyroxine

   D. Clonidine

   E. None of the above

284. MAOI is contraindicated in which of the following medical conditions?

   A. Hepatic disease

   B. CHF

   C. Pheochromocytoma

   D. Renal impairment

   E. All of the above

285. Which of the following is true regarding the mechanism of VPA's teratogenicity?

   A. Inhibition of the enzyme dihydrofolate reductase

   B. Formation of free radicals during microsomal metabolism of VPA

   C. Inhibition of thymidylate synthase

   D. Inhibition of colony-stimulating factor

   E. All of the above

286. All of the following statements accurately describe the neuromolecular effects of asenapine EXCEPT:

 A. Antagonism at serotonergic receptor

 B. Antagonism at dopaminergic receptor

 C. Antagonism at muscarinic receptors

 D. Antagonism at adrenergic receptor

 E. Partial agonist at 5-HT$_2$A receptor

287. Which of the following benzodiazepines is used as an adjuvant to lithium in the treatment of mania?

 A. Temazepam

 B. Flurazepam

 C. Clonazepam

 D. Diazepam

 E. All of the above

288. All of the following conditions can mimic NMS EXCEPT:

 A. Environmental heatstroke

 B. Serotonin syndrome

 C. Withdrawal from dopamine agonists

 D. Malignant hyperthermia

 E. None of the above

289. Which of the following is associated with VPA exposure during pregnancy?

    A. Hepatotoxicity

    B. Coagulopathies

    C. Neonatal hypoglycemia

    D. Neural tube defects

    E. All of the above

290. Most adverse effects of carbamazepine are correlated with which of the following plasma concentration?

    A. >4 μg per ml

    B. >6 μg per ml

    C. >9 μg per ml

    D. >15 μg per ml

    E. None of the above

291. Genetic polymorphisms in the cytochrome genes can code for inefficient versions of cytochrome enzymes leading to impaired drug metabolism (poor metabolizers). Which of the following ethnic groups carry the highest percentage of poor metabolizers of the CYP2D6 isoenzyme?

    A. Whites

    B. Asians

    C. African Americans

    D. Native Americans

    E. None of the above

292. The pentobarbital challenge test is used to

    A. Guide detoxification from barbiturates

    B. Diagnose intermittent porphyria

    C. Determine dose for "amytal interview"

    D. Determine dosing for treatment refractory tonic-clonic seizures

    E. Diagnose asthma

293. All of the following are true regarding lithium EXCEPT:

    A. Lithium is excreted unchanged by the kidney

    B. Lithium is not metabolized by the liver

    C. Lithium has mild proserotonergic and adrenergic effects

    D. Lithium is a naturally occurring cation

    E. None of the above

294. A 49-year-old woman with breast cancer is currently taking tamoxifen. She develops depressive symptoms and is referred to a psychiatrist. She meets the criteria for major depressive disorder. Which of the following medications interacts with tamoxifen?

    A. SJW

    B. Paroxetine

    C. Duloxetine

    D. Sertraline

    E. All of the above

295. Which of the following drugs has shown to cause the most QTc prolongation at therapeutic doses?

 A. Olanzapine

 B. Thioridazine

 C. Haloperidol

 D. Ziprasidone

 E. Risperidone

296. Which of the following drugs has none to minimal interactions with the cytochrome isoenzymes?

 A. Desvenlafaxine

 B. Atomoxetine

 C. Modafinil

 D. Duloxetine

 E. All of the above

297. Which of the following properties of pindolol supports its use as an augmentation agent in the treatment of depression?

 A. Selective β-adrenergic antagonistic effects

 B. Nonselective β-adrenergic antagonistic effects

 C. Sympathomimetic effects

 D. α-Adrenergic and β-adrenergic antagonistic effect

 E. All of the above

298. All of the following are antipsychotic-induced adverse effects related to dopamine antagonism EXCEPT:

    A. Galactorrhea

    B. NMS

    C. Premature ejaculation

    D. Bone loss

    E. None of the above

299. The CATIE trial, which included 1,493 participants from 57 US institutions, concluded that the greatest body weight gain was observed with which of the following antipsychotics?

    A. Olanzapine

    B. Ziprasidone

    C. Quetiapine

    D. Risperidone

    E. Perphenazine

300. Which of the following is true regarding cardiac side effects during treatment with therapeutic levels of lithium?

    A. Nonspecific T wave changes

    B. Prolonged QTc

    C. ST depression

    D. Torsades de pointes

    E. None of the above

301. Which of the following is teratogenic effect of carbamazepine?

    A. Fingernail hypoplasia

    B. Spina bifida

    C. Craniofacial abnormalities

    D. Inguinal hernia

    E. All of the above

302. What is the rate of Ebstein anomaly with lithium-exposed neonates?

    A. 1% to 2%

    B. 0.1% to 0.7%

    C. 2% to 3%

    D. 2% to 3.5%

    E. None of the above

303. You manage care of a depressed patient with a history of epilepsy who is currently on a VPA, which is also a substrate for CYP system. Which of the following antidepressants would be most appropriate for use in this patient from the standpoint of not increasing the risk of seizures?

    A. Phenelzine

    B. Maprotiline

    C. Clomipramine

    D. Bupropion

    E. Fluoxetine

304. A 50-year-old man with a history of treatment refractory depression is started on phenelzine. He is gradually titrated to a daily dose of 30 mg. He complains of frequent dizzy spells. You decrease the dose of phenelzine and ask him to increase his dietary sodium intake. Despite these measures, he continues to experience orthostatic hypotension. You decide to switch him over to tranylcypromine. Which of the following dosing strategies should you use?

A. Discontinue phenelzine and start tranylcypromine immediately

B. Taper phenelzine while starting tranylcypromine

C. Discontinue phenelzine, wait for 2 weeks, and then start tranylcypromine

D. Discontinue phenelzine, wait for 4 weeks, and then start tranylcypromine

E. None of the above

305. Which of the following antipsychotic medications when given orally causes the least QTc prolongation at therapeutic doses?

A. Risperidone

B. Quetiapine

C. Haloperidol

D. Ziprasidone

E. Olanzapine

306. Which of the following antidepressant medications is most useful in the treatment refractory of an anergic depressed patient?

A. Mirtazapine

B. Tranylcypromine

C. Citalopram

D. Paroxetine

E. Nortriptyline

307. A 26-year-old 16-week postpartum African American woman presents with low mood for the past 6 weeks. She reports no interest in life and cannot enjoy her adorable 4-month-old baby girl. She stopped nursing about 6 weeks ago but is able to care for her. She reports her husband as very supportive. She sleeps only 3 hours a day and has no energy. She denies changes in her psychomotor activity levels although she has to push herself to get things accomplished. She lost 20 lb (9 kg) in 4 weeks because of decreased appetite. She denies suicidal or homicidal ideation, and there is no evidence of psychosis. Which of the following would be the most appropriate medication to start?

    A. Fluoxetine

    B. Mirtazapine

    C. Aripiprazole

    D. Bupropion

    E. Venlafaxine

308. Which of the following is true regarding vilazodone?

    A. It is partial agonist at 5-HT$_1$A receptor

    B. The drug's bioavailability is unchanged with coadministration of food

    C. It is a dual serotonin–norepinephrine reuptake inhibitor (SNRI)

    D. It is an FDA-approved treatment for GAD

    E. The recommended dose of vilazodone is 80 mg once daily

309. Which of following TCAs has most antihistaminergic activity?

    A. Nortriptyline

    B. Desipramine

    C. Doxepin

    D. Amoxapine

    E. Protriptyline

310. Which of following pharmacologic agents used in treatment of insomnia has the shortest half-life?

    A. Temazepam

    B. Zaleplon

    C. Eszopiclone

    D. Trazodone

    E. Triazolam

311. Which of following SSRIs is most likely to cause a discontinuation syndrome?

    A. Citalopram

    B. Fluoxetine

    C. Sertraline

    D. Paroxetine

    E. Fluvoxamine

312. You are treating a 53-year-old man with chronic schizoaffective disorder with combination of olanzapine 10 mg a day, venlafaxine 225 mg once daily, clonazepam 1 mg twice daily, and trazodone 150 mg at bedtime. The patient returns to the office for routine follow-up visit and complains of pathologic crying. He states that he has uncontrolled crying triggered by minor or no stimulus. He is unable to watch television and has difficulty interacting with family members. He reports these symptoms being present for the due past 2 to 3 weeks. He denies any change in his medications. On further inquiry, he also reports some gait instability, dizziness and lightheadedness, electric shock-like sensation, and muscle spasm. Brief neurologic examination is negative. Which of the following interventions would be most appropriate at this stage?

    A. Obtain a urine drug screening

    B. Start workup for TIA or stroke

    C. Increase dose of olanzapine

    D. Carefully review pharmacy refill records for possible medication noncompliance

    E. Augment with divalproex sodium

313. Which of following endocrine side effects is most commonly seen with lithium therapy?

   A. Hyperthyroidism

   B. Hypothyroidism

   C. Hypoparathyroidism

   D. Hypocalcemia

   E. Hypoglycemia

314. A 27-year-old woman comes to you with complains of mood swings, anger, anxiety, irritability, and bloating at time of menstruation. Which of following medications could be used in her treatment?

   A. Bupropion

   B. Mirtazapine

   C. Paroxetine

   D. Aripiprazole

   E. Clonazepam

315. A 30-year-old Caucasian woman comes to you complaining of excessive sleep, increasing apathy, and increasing eating habits. She also reports that she is more irritable and there are days where she goes without sleep. Three months ago she spent almost $500 on buying clothes and $1,000 on electronics. About a year ago when she experienced similar symptoms, she saw her family care physician who prescribed fluoxetine that made her very jittery, and she did not sleep for many days. Which of the following medications will be most appropriate in her management?

   A. Paroxetine

   B. Mirtazapine

   C. Lithium carbonate

   D. Clonazepam

   E. Topiramate

316. A 32-year-old veteran is being treated for PTSD. He recently started taking a new medication for his nightmares and insomnia. After few days, he comes into the emergency department with complaints of prolonged and painful erection. The emergency physician asks him to discontinue one of his medications. Which of the following medications is the cause of the patient's presentation?

    A. Mirtazapine

    B. Citalopram

    C. Zolpidem

    D. Prazosin

    E. Temazepam

317. A 35-year-old man with a history of bipolar depression is brought to the emergency department by his friends. The patient was found unresponsive. Patient is minimally responsive in the emergency department, and he complains of dry mouth and blurred vision. On examination, he has dilated pupils, and cardiac monitoring shows premature ventricular contractions and tachycardia about 140 beats per minute. Preliminary diagnosis of a drug overdose is presumed. Which of following medications is most likely to be involved in his overdose?

    A. Paroxetine

    B. Venlafaxine

    C. Nortriptyline

    D. Mirtazapine

    E. Divalproex sodium

318. You are treating a 54-year-old man for panic disorder with agoraphobia. He is taking citalopram 40 mg once daily and trazodone 100 mg at bedtime for insomnia. He is requesting a medication to control his panic attacks. You decide to prescribe him benzodiazepine. Which of following benzodiazepines has a high risk of withdrawal symptoms including life-threatening seizures?

    A. Alprazolam

    B. Chlordiazepoxide

    C. Temazepam

    D. Clonazepam

    E. Diazepam

319. Which of following mood stabilizers carries the risk of worsening psoriasis?

    A. Topiramate

    B. Lithium carbonate

    C. Risperidone

    D. Clonazepam

    E. Aripiprazole

320. Which of the following atypical neuroleptic agents is known to have the least extrapyramidal side effects?

    A. Olanzapine

    B. Clozapine

    C. Aripiprazole

    D. Ziprasidone

    E. Risperidone

321. All of the following statements are true regarding SSRIs EXCEPT:

    A. Higher doses are required to treat OCD

    B. SSRIs have a flat dose–response curve

    C. It is safe to use a different SSRI on a patient with a history of allergy to one SSRI

    D. Premenstrual dysphoric disorder (PMDD) responds well to SSRI treatment during late luteal phase

    E. None of the above

322. A 32-year-old Caucasian man with schizophrenia was discharged from an inpatient unit 3 days ago. He is known for his noncompliance with his treatment, and currently, he is stabilized on risperidone-injection (Risperdal Consta) IM every 2 weeks. He is also on risperidone 3 mg twice a day orally. Which of the following statements should be taken into consideration before stopping the oral risperidone?

    A. Risperidone microspheres start releasing significant amount of drug, 3 weeks after the injection

    B. When dose adjustment is made, clinical effects are expected after 3 weeks, following the injection at higher dose

    C. Maximal drug release occurs after 5 weeks

    D. Oral therapy should be continued for 3 weeks after the onset of IM therapy

    E. All of the above

323. Which of the following is/are true regarding drug interactions with olanzapine extended release injectable suspension?

    A. Carbamazepine increases the clearance of olanzapine

    B. Fluvoxamine might increase olanzapine levels

    C. VPA may result in decreased olanzapine plasma concentrations

    D. Injections are only for IM use and should not be given intravenously

    E. All of the above

324. Administration of SJW can decrease contraceptive efficacy by which of the following mechanisms of action?

    A. Inducing the CYP3A4 isoenzyme

    B. Inducing the CYP2D6 isoenzyme

    C. Inducing the glycoprotein transport across intestinal lumen

    D. Inhibiting the CYP3A4 isoenzyme

    E. All of the above

325. Which of the following conventional antipsychotics is designated as high potency?

    A. Thioridazine

    B. Chlorpromazine

    C. Pimozide

    D. Mesoridazine

    E. Perphenazine

326. Which of the following statements is/are true regarding the treatment of eating disorder?

    A. No pharmacotherapy is proven to be efficacious for anorexia nervosa

    B. Calorie and psychotherapy are proven to be efficacious for anorexia nervosa

    C. SSRIs are the first-line treatment for bulimia nervosa

    D. First-line treatment for binge eating disorder is uncertain

    E. All of the above

327. Ms. C, a 53-year-old Caucasian woman suffers from an autosomal dominant neurodegenerative disorder. She is presenting to your clinic with motor, cognitive, and psychiatric symptoms. Her genetic testing confirms CAG repeats. Which of the following medications is approved by FDA for the treatment of her involuntary motor movements?

    A. Olanzapine

    B. Haloperidol

    C. Fluoxetine

    D. Tetrabenazine

    E. Clonazepam

328. Which of the following is used in the management of neuroleptic-induced dystonia?

    A. Phencyclidine

    B. Propranolol

    C. Benztropine

    D. Phenobarbital

    E. All of the above

329. Which of the following psychotropic medications increases the metabolism of oral contraceptive pills resulting in decreased efficacy of birth control?

    A. Carbamazepine

    B. SJW

    C. Modafinil

    D. Topiramate

    E. All of the above

330. Which of the following agents can be used in the treatment of premature ejaculation?

    A. Desipramine

    B. Lorazepam

    C. Fluoxetine

    D. Mirtazapine

    E. Phenelzine

331. Which of the following medications selectively inhibits MAO-A?

    A. Isocarboxazid

    B. Phenelzine

    C. Selegiline

    D. Moclobemide

    E. Tranylcypromine

332. By measuring their plasma drug levels, all of the following psychotropic agents may be clinically useful for optimal efficacious dosing EXCEPT:

    A. Lithium

    B. VPA

    C. Nortriptyline

    D. Lamotrigine

    E. Clozapine

333. Which of the following is true regarding prolactin level during neuro-leptic therapy?

    A. Risperidone increases the prolactin level the most among the atypical neuroleptics

    B. Clozapine has the least effect on prolactin therapy

    C. Aripiprazole can be used to normalize neuroleptic-induced pro-lactin elevation

    D. Typical antipsychotics are associated with persistently elevated prolactin level

    E. All of the above

334. A 46-year-old Caucasian man is being treated for major depressive dis-order, which is currently in remission for about a year now. He has had three episodes of depression over his lifetime, and his last psychiatric hospitalization was about 3 years ago for a suicide attempt. He has also had chronic back pain. His partner expresses concern about his ongo-ing antidepressant therapy and asks if and when he can stop his anti-depressants. Which of the following is the most appropriate statement regarding his management?

    A. Antidepressant therapy can be safely discontinued after 6 months of remission of his depressive symptoms

    B. Antidepressant therapy can be safely discontinued after 12 months of remission of his depressive symptoms

    C. Antidepressant therapy can be safely discontinued provided patient agrees to monthly maintenance ECTs

    D. Lifelong antidepressant maintenance treatment is indicated for this patient

    E. A drug holiday of at least 3 months must be attempted before considering antidepressant discontinuation in this patient

335. Which of the following medications can be used for the treatment of GAD that is not sedating?

   A. Alprazolam

   B. Clonazepam

   C. Paroxetine

   D. Buspirone

   E. Mirtazapine

336. Mr. A overdosed on scopolamine prescribed for his motion sickness. Which of the following can be used in treating scopolamine overdose?

   A. Phentolamine

   B. Physostigmine

   C. Atropine

   D. Diphenhydramine

   E. Flumazenil

337. Concurrent administration of all of the following medications may increase the concentration of lamotrigine EXCEPT:

   A. Fluoxetine

   B. Alprazolam

   C. Bupropion

   D. Oral contraceptive pills

   E. VPA

338. A 43-year-old combat veteran with PTSD complains of frequent night-mares. His partner expresses concerns that he wakes up in the middle of the night screaming. You started him on prazosin with significant benefit. His medical condition is significant for chronic pain for which he is on amitriptyline. He was commenced on vardenafil for his erectile dysfunction by his PCP. Which of the following side effect would you expect as a result of DDI between vardenafil and prazosin?

A. Sexual side effects

B. Drowsiness

C. Hypotension

D. Urinary retention

E. Priapism

339. All of the following are true regarding lithium EXCEPT:

A. Hemodialysis is indicated for lithium overdose presenting with neurotoxicity

B. Patients on lithium should reduce their sodium intake

C. Current recommendation is to measure lithium level after 6 months

D. Serum lithium level should be measured in the sample drawn after 12 hours of the last dose

E. History of good functioning between episodes predicts a positive response to lithium prophylaxis

340. A 39-year-old schizophrenic man was hospitalized on a locked psychiatric unit for worsening hallucinations and paranoia. He was stabilized on olanzapine 10 mg every day and was discharged home. You see him in the clinic 3 weeks after discharge. He reports hearing voices again. His wife confirms medication compliance. You note a trial of bupropion in his discharge summary to address his nicotine dependence. On enquiry, you find out that the patient resumed smoking after a brief period of abstinence when he was hospitalized. Which of the following is the most likely cause of his relapse?

   A. Bupropion-induced psychosis
   B. Treatment-resistant schizophrenia
   C. Antipsychotic noncompliance
   D. Antipsychotic–smoking CYP-mediated interaction
   E. None of the above

341. Which of the following atypical antipsychotics is associated with least weight gain according to the CATIE trial?

   A. Olanzapine
   B. Ziprasidone
   C. Quetiapine
   D. Risperidone
   E. Perphenazine

342. Concurrent administration of triazolam and which of the following results in triazolam toxicity?

   A. Nefazodone
   B. Ketoconazole
   C. Amprenavir
   D. Efavirenz
   E. All of the above

343. Phentolamine is the treatment of choice for which of the following conditions?

    A. Serotonin syndrome

    B. Malignant hyperthermia

    C. NMS

    D. Hypertensive crisis associated with MAOI and tyramine ingestion

    E. Catatonia

344. Thioridazine is associated with which of the following side effects?

    A. Retrograde ejaculation

    B. Torsades de pointes

    C. Agranulocytosis

    D. Retinal pigmentation

    E. All of the above

345. A 47-year-old Caucasian man is admitted to medical department for nausea and vomiting of 5 days duration. His past medical history is significant for obesity. He does not have past psychiatric history. He suddenly developed focal neck muscle spasm. His chin is turned to one side with his head turned to the other side. Which of the following nonpsychiatric medications could have caused his acute focal dystonia?

    A. Propranolol

    B. Metoclopramide

    C. Diphenhydramine

    D. Meclizine

    E. All of the above

346. Which of the following antidepressants would be the most appropriate choice in the management of depression after MI?

    A. Venlafaxine

    B. Nortriptyline

    C. Sertraline

    D. Fluvoxamine

    E. Phenelzine

347. Which of the following is recommended for the treatment of depression with psychotic features?

    A. Monotherapy with antidepressant

    B. Combination of an antidepressant and a mood stabilizer

    C. Combination of an antidepressant and an antipsychotic

    D. Combination of an antidepressant and psychotherapy

    E. Combination of an antipsychotic and psychotherapy

348. Which of the following agents is the treatment of choice for psychosis in Parkinson disease?

    A. Ziprasidone

    B. Olanzapine

    C. Quetiapine

    D. Risperidone

    E. Haloperidol

349. A 39-year-old Caucasian man with suspected nosocomial pneumonia caused by *S. aureus* is admitted to medical department. The primary team consults you for the management of his worsening anxiety and nightmares. You interview the patient and find out that he has been diagnosed with combat-related PTSD and is currently taking a combination of clonidine, trazodone, and ziprasidone for his symptoms. You also note the infectious disease consultation recommending treatment with the antibiotic linezolid. You should warn the primary team to watch out for which of the following DDIs?

  A. Muscle cramps, excessive salivation, and diaphoresis

  B. Hyperthermia, dizziness, and diarrhea

  C. Muscle rigidity, hyperthermia, and altered mental status

  D. Ataxia and tremor

  E. Visual hallucination

350. Which of the following agents is contraindicated in the treatment of mixed overdose with tricyclics and benzodiazepine?

  A. Sodium bicarbonate

  B. IV fluids

  C. Flumazenil

  D. Naloxone

  E. None of the above

351. Which of the following statements regarding oxcarbazepine is true?

  A. Oxcarbazepine offers significant advantage about enzyme induction and autoinduction when compared with carbamazepine

  B. Hypernatremia is a concern with oxcarbazepine therapy

  C. Oxcarbazepine has a lower risk of hematologic events (e.g., pancytopenia, agranulocytosis, and leukopenia) compared with carbamazepine

  D. All of the above

  E. None of the above

352. Concurrent use of risperidone and the lipid-lowering agent simvastatin can lead to which of the following clinical scenarios?

    A. Increased risk of myopathy

    B. Reduction in the cholesterol-lowering effectiveness of simvastatin

    C. Increased risk of extrapyramidal symptoms (EPS)

    D. Lower serum risperidone concentrations and necessitate an increase in dose of risperidone

    E. Additive cognitive side effects

353. Which of the following antidepressants is devoid of sexual side effects?

    A. Nefazodone

    B. Paroxetine

    C. Venlafaxine

    D. Duloxetine

    E. Escitalopram

354. You are managing a 30-year-old man patient on a chemical dependency unit who is diagnosed with bipolar affective disorder and alcohol dependence. He is sober for the 30 days. His family history is significant for bipolar disorder in his mother. He added that she is responding well to Depakote (VPA) and he wants to try it. Liver function tests and CBC are normal. After educating the patient about the risk of Depakote-induced pancreatitis, on which of the following issues should you lay emphasis while agreeing to start Depakote?

    A. Abstinence from alcohol during the course of Depakote therapy

    B. Compliance with laboratory testing for serum amylase every 3 months

    C. Immediately reporting symptoms such as ankle swelling and shortness of breath

    D. Sleeplessness

    E. Avoiding foods with high fat content

    F. All of the above

355. All of the following antipsychotic agents have potential to increase prolactin levels EXCEPT:

    A. Risperidone

    B. Ziprasidone

    C. Aripiprazole

    D. Paliperidone

    E. Quetiapine

356. Which of the following is not true of antipsychotic-induced weight gain?

    A. Rapid weight gain within the few months of treatment

    B. Antipsychotic-induced weight gain is solely correlated to the affinity of the antipsychotic drug for histamine receptors

    C. Currently approved pharmacologic treatments for obesity lack clear evidence of efficacy and safety in managing antipsychotic-induced weight gain

    D. Antipsychotic-induced weight gain is best managed by diet, exercise, and behavioral interventions

    E. A combination of antipsychotic-induced weight gain and insulin sensitivity contributes to the increased risk of diabetes in schizophrenia

357. Which of the following mood stabilizers can be safely used in the treatment of bipolar disorder in a patient with past medical history significant for liver cirrhosis?

    A. Lithium

    B. Carbamazepine

    C. Olanzapine

    D. VPA

    E. All of the above

358. All the following statements regarding low platelet counts and thrombocytopenia associated with VPA therapy are true EXCEPT:

  A. The mechanism of VPA-induced thrombocytopenia is believed to be an immune destruction of platelets by VPA

  B. The risk of VPA-induced thrombocytopenia is dose related

  C. Elderly patients, women, and those with low baseline platelet counts appear to be at higher risk for VPA-induced thrombocytopenia

  D. It is not uncommon to see a drop in platelet count without thrombocytopenia or adverse clinical events in psychiatric patients receiving VPA

  E. VPA-induced low platelet counts can be managed by close monitoring and may resolve without interruption of VPA treatment

359. Topiramate is useful in all of the following clinical conditions EXCEPT:

  A. Seizure

  B. Migraine prophylaxis

  C. Eating disorder

  D. Alcohol dependence

  E. Bipolar disorder, manic episode

360. Which of the following is the most common side effect of SSRIs?

  A. GI

  B. Sexual side effect

  C. Weight gain

  D. Insomnia

  E. Abnormal dreams

361. Which of the following SSRIs has dopaminergic activity?

   A. Fluvoxamine

   B. Sertraline

   C. Fluoxetine

   D. Citalopram

   E. None of the above

362. All of the following are FDA-approved indications for aripiprazole EXCEPT:

   A. Bipolar disorder, depressed phase

   B. Bipolar disorder, manic phase

   C. Autistic disorder, psychomotor agitation

   D. Schizophrenia

   E. Adjunctive treatment in major depressive disorder (MDD)

363. Which of the following antipsychotics is approved as a monotherapy for bipolar depression?

   A. Ziprasidone

   B. Aripiprazole

   C. Olanzapine

   D. Quetiapine

   E. Lurasidone

364. In which of the following psychiatric conditions can the therapeutic lag with SSRIs be as long as 8 to 12 weeks?

   A. MDD

   B. GAD

   C. PTSD

   D. PMDD

   E. Bulimia nervosa

365. Which of the following psychotropics is associated with sialorrhea?

    A. Nortriptyline

    B. Paroxetine

    C. Aripiprazole

    D. Clozapine

    E. Lithium

366. Which is the following SSRIs has the most affinity to muscarinic receptors?

    A. Citalopram

    B. Sertraline

    C. Fluoxetine

    D. Fluvoxamine

    E. Paroxetine

367. Which of the following class of drugs has been associated with the development of a frontal lobe type syndrome characterized by apathy, indifference, loss of initiative, and/or disinhibition?

    A. SSRIs

    B. Atypical antipsychotics

    C. Stimulants

    D. Anticonvulsant mood stabilizers

    E. Cognitive enhancers

Answers

1. **Answer: B.** Amitriptyline

   Combined MAOI–TCA therapy is safe, provided if you add MAOI to an established tricylic regimen. The other agents listed are contraindicated, and they can cause life-threatening serotonin syndrome when combined with MAOIs.

2. **Answer: B.** 2 weeks

   With the irreversible nonselective MAOIs (phenelzine and tranylcypromine), it takes up to 2 weeks to regenerate normal levels of MAOI, whereas, with the reversible selective MAOI (moclobemide), there is prompt restoration of metabolically active levels of MAO enzymes after discontinuation.

3. **Answer: B.** Mirtazapine

   Mirtazapine antagonizes central presynaptic α_2-adrenergic receptors leading to increased release of serotonin and norepinephrine in the synaptic cleft. Mirtazapine is effective in the treatment of PTSD. Prazosin inhibits central postsynaptic α-adrenergic receptor, whereas clonidine is a central α-adrenergic receptor agonist. Venlafaxine is an SNRI, whereas naltrexone is an opioid receptor antagonist. All the aforementioned agents except naltrexone are useful in the management of PTSD.

4. **Answer: B.** Weight gain

   Weight gain is a common side effect associated with mirtazapine. Other common side effects include dizziness, drowsiness, sedation, malaise, and erectile dysfunction. Hyponatremia is a side effect of SSRI therapy. Hepatic toxicity is associated with anticonvulsants and several psychotropic agents such as nefazodone, tacrine, vanishing bile duct syndrome in chlorpromazine, and haloperidol, but it is not associated with mirtazapine. Clozapine and carbamazepine have the highest incidence of agranulocytosis among the psychotropics even though other psychotropics are increasingly reported to cause hematologic abnormalities.

5. **Answer: A.** Clozapine improves negative symptoms in schizophrenia

Clozapine is effective in treatment-resistant schizophrenia and improves negative symptoms. There is evidence for clozapine in treatment-resistant mania. Clozapine can cause NMS, although the presentation may be different from that of traditional antipsychotics. Clozapine-induced NMS is less likely to manifest with extrapyramidal features such as rigidity and tremor. The incidence of clozapine-induced agranulocytosis is between 1% and 2%.

6. **Answer: A.** Bupropion

Unlike other antidepressants, bupropion may shorten REM latency and increase total REM sleep. SSRIs, TCAs, and MAOIs generally suppress REM sleep.

7. **Answer: D.** Molindone

Molindone is an intermediate potency conventional antipsychotic that tends to decrease appetite and even cause weight loss. The atypical antipsychotics listed are associated with either weight neutral or modest weight gain.

8. **Answer: A.** Alprazolam

There is some evidence for effectiveness of alprazolam in the treatment of mild to moderate major depressive disorder. α-Interferon (used in the treatment of hepatitis C), propranolol (β-adrenergic blocker), varenicline (partial agonist at the nicotinic receptor and used for tobacco cessation), and depot-medroxyprogesterone acetate (hormonal contraceptive) can lead to mood problems.

9. **Answer: B.** Hyporeflexia

Hyperreflexia, and not hyporeflexia, is common in serotonin syndrome. The presence of myoclonus distinguishes serotonin syndrome from NMS. Serotonin neurons play a role in thermoregulation; an increase in serotonergic activity can lead to thermoregulatory dysfunction that explains the fever and shivering seen in serotonin syndrome.

10. Answer: E. All of the above   NE

Amoxapine is noradrenergic TCA. Amoxapine causes extrapyramidal side effects because of its dopamine blocking activity. It is FDA approved for reactive depressive disorder, psychotic depression, and depression accompanied by anxiety or agitation. In cases of overdose, cardiac arrhythmias and seizures are seen possibly because of blockade of ion channels.

11. Answer: A. Fluphenazine

Fluphenazine belongs to the piperazine–phenothiazine class of antipsychotics. The drug has minimal α-adrenergic blocking effect and thus is less likely to cause postural hypotension.

12. Answer: B. Order a thyroid-stimulating hormone (TSH) level

The incidence of goiter and hypothyroidism during lithium therapy is 40% and 20%, respectively. Dry skin, hair loss, cold intolerance, fatigue, constipation, and depression are some symptoms of hypothyroidism. Diagnoses and management of endocrine abnormalities must be attempted before discontinuing lithium therapy. Abrupt discontinuing of lithium can trigger significant relapses.

13. Answer: D. Fluoxetine

According to *Diagnostic and Statistical Manual of Mental Disorders* (Fourth Edition) criteria, patients with body dysmorphic disorder (BDD) who lack insight, who have referential thinking, and who have very fixed delusions are double coded with a diagnosis of BDD as well as delusional disorder, somatic type. Fluoxetine, an SSRI, is the recommended treatment of this condition. Although antipsychotics may sound like a logical choice for these patients, there is more evidence for the safety and efficacy of fluoxetine compared with antipsychotic monotherapy in delusional and nondelusional patients with BDD.

14. **Answer: A.** Carbamazepine

Carbamazepine is structurally similar to TCAs, and hence, it should be avoided in cases of known hypersensitivity to any of the TCAs.

15. **Answer: B.** Discontinue clozapine immediately and monitor WBC and ANC for 4 weeks

After discontinuation of clozapine, monitor WBC and ANC for at least 4 weeks from day of discontinuation until they normalize. The following schedule is recommended: daily until WBC count >3,000 per mm^3 and ANC >1,500 per mm^3, twice weekly until WBC count >3,500 per mm^3 and ANC >2,000 per mm^3, and weekly after WBC count >3,500 per mm^3.

16. **Answer: B.** Inhibition of the enzyme carbonic anhydrase

Topiramate, a carbonic anhydrase inhibitor, can lead to metabolic acidosis, hypercalciuria, and elevated urine pH, thus posing an increased risk of calcium phosphate renal stones.

17. **Answer: C.** The patient will need an increased dose of the extended release formulation to maintain therapeutic VPA levels

The bioavailability of divalproex-enteric coated (ER) is approximately 10% less than that of the delayed-release tablets. An 8% to 20% higher divalproex-ER daily dose should be considered while converting from divalproex-EC to divalproex-ER. The side effect profiles of both formulations are the same.

18. **Answer: A.** Maintenance doses of lithium are given three times weekly at the beginning of each dialysis session

Lithium is dialyzable and hence should be administered immediately after dialysis. Lithium circulates unchanged in the body between dialysis sessions, and lithium levels during dialysis are usually drawn 2 to 3 hours post dose. Monthly lithium level is recommended because dialysis patients experience fluid shifts.

19. **Answer: B.** Possibility of side effects because of the presence of nonidentical inactive ingredients in the generic version

Although the active ingredient is the same, the inactive ingredients in generic medications are usually different. These nonidentical inactive ingredients can cause unusual or allergic side effects. Although there have been reports of altered bioavailability between the brand and generic formulations of clozapine, the clinical significance of these differences is not well established. Currently, there is no evidence that switching the patients to generic formulation poses an increased risk of agranulocytosis.

20. **Answer: C.** Baseline, 12 weeks, and annually

The monitoring protocol for patients on atypical antipsychotics includes fasting plasma glucose at baseline, 12 weeks, and then annually. This should be done more frequently in patients with a higher baseline risk for diabetes.

21. **Answer: B.** *O*-desmethylvenlafaxine

Venlafaxine is an SNRI. *O*-desmethylvenlafaxine (active metabolite of venlafaxine) is formed by polymorphic isoenzyme CYP2D6. Like venlafaxine, *O*-desmethylvenlafaxine inhibits the reuptake of both serotonin and norepinephrine. It also has a weak inhibitory effects on the reuptake of dopamine receptors. *N*-desmethylvenlafaxine (less pharmacologically active) is formed by CYP3A4. Both *O*-desmethylvenlafaxine and *N*-desmethylvenlafaxine are converted into *N,O*-didesmethylvenlafaxine (less pharmacologically active).

22. **Answer: E.** Moderate interaction with the CYP system

Desvenlafaxine has minimal interaction with the CYP isoenzymes. This may reduce potential DDIs. No titration is required while starting the recommended dose. Side effects occur in the first week of therapy and resolve soon. Most common side effect is nausea. GI side effects may be more frequent in women than in men, and educating the patients helps in achieving compliance.

23. **Answer: B.** Old age is a major risk factor

Neuroleptic-induced acute dystonia occurs frequently in young men. Risk factors are prior dystonic reactions to neuroleptic agents and the use of high-potency typical neuroleptic medication. The signs or symptoms start within 7 days of initiating or rapidly raising the dose of neuroleptic medication or of reducing anticholinergic agents. Generally, neuroleptic-induced acute dystonia is not seen with clozapine therapy. Tardive dystonia occurs with prolonged exposure to antipsychotics. It is characterized by sustained muscle contractions, repetitive movements, or abnormal postures. Tardive dystonia responds well to clozapine.

24. **Answer: B.** Serotonin (5-HT$_1$A) receptors

Buspirone acts on 5-HT$_1$A receptors. The anxiolytic property of buspirone possibly results from the partial agonist actions at postsynaptic region by reducing serotonergic activity. The antidepressant effect is a result of partial agonistic action at presynaptic serotonin autoreceptors and by increasing the serotonergic activity. Buspirone is also a D$_2$ agonist and antagonist. It does not act at α_2-adrenergic, GABA$_A$, or muscarinic receptors.

25. **Answer: E.** All of the above

NMS is a life-threatening complication of antipsychotic drug use. Clinical manifestations of NMS are hyperthermia, severe EPS, and autonomic dysfunction. Prior episodes of NMS, affective disorder, dehydration, high doses of neuroleptic medication, rapid increase in dosage, and IM injection of neuroleptic medication are risk factors for NMS. The risk for recurrence on reexposure to neuroleptic is approximately 30%, and the risk is high during the first month. Recurrence of NMS may be minimized by delaying rechallenge by 2 weeks post NMS.

26. **Answer: C.** Bupropion

Among the listed choices, both mirtazapine and bupropion have little or no sexual side effects. However, mirtazapine causes weight gain. Fluoxetine causes sexual side effects. Bupropion and fluoxetine do not cause weight gain and, in fact, do cause weight loss. Nortriptyline and paroxetine cause both sexual side effects and weight gain.

27. **Answer: B.** Plasma levels >350 ng per ml

Plasma clozapine levels >350 ng per ml suggests efficacious dosage. A therapeutic range of clozapine serum levels is not recognized. However, if there is no clinical response after optimal dosing (450 mg per day) in 6 weeks, serum levels should be measured.

28. **Answer: D.** Nephrogenic diabetes insipidus

Nephrogenic diabetes insipidus is characterized by polydipsia and polyuria (up to 20 L per day). Carbamazepine causes SIADH and not nephrogenic diabetes insipidus.

29. **Answer: A.** Pancreatitis

Sedation, nausea, weight gain, hand tremors, reversible elevations in liver enzymes, and transient elevations in blood ammonia levels are some of the dose-related side effects.

30. **Answer: E.** All of the above

Prospective studies have indicated that clozapine appears to be an effective pharmacotherapy for severe water imbalance in schizophrenia. Clozapine is efficacious in treatment-resistant schizophrenia and improves negative symptoms. There is evidence for clozapine in treatment-resistant mania, reducing hostility and aggression.

31. **Answer: D.** Chloride

Barbiturates, benzodiazepine, and nonbenzodiazepine hypnotic drugs are positive allosteric modulators of the $GABA_A$-receptor complex. By binding to a distinct site on the receptor, they increase chloride conductance.

32. **Answer: B.** Benztropine

Benztropine has least abuse potential. There is evidence for abuse potential with trihexyphenidyl, diphenhydramine, and scopolamine. Benzhexol (trihexyphenidyl) is the most abused anticholinergic agent, and other popular anticholinergics are orphenadrine and biperiden. Procyclidine also has less abuse potential.

33. **Answer: D.** Serum concentration of VPA should not exceed 150 μg per ml

Neonatal risks may be reduced by maintaining serum concentration <70 μg per ml. Folate should be administered throughout the gestation, and vitamin K supplementation should be considered during the last month of gestation.

34. **Answer: A.** Depression is associated with increased REM density, although temazepam has no effect on REM sleep

Depression is associated with increased REM density. Temazepam has no effect on REM sleep but increases stage II sleep.

35. **Answer: E.** All of the above

Like benzodiazepines and barbiturates, both clonidine and guanfacine can cause discontinuation symptoms.

36. **Answer: B.** Clonidine

Clonidine, methyldopa, and guanfacine are α_2-adrenergic agonists. Yohimbine is an α_2-adrenergic receptor antagonist. Reserpine is a dopamine receptor antagonist and a centrally acting adrenergic neuron blocker. Mirtazapine is an α_2-adrenergic antagonist.

37. **Answer: B.** Check his lithium level, and in a week, contact him with the results

The appropriate action is to check the lithium level. Reducing the dose of lithium to 1,000 mg or increasing the paroxetine to 30 mg is not recommended. Concurrent use of paroxetine and lithium may increase the risk of serotonin syndrome and may increase serum lithium concentration. There is no need for dose changes when his affective symptoms are stable, and there are no signs of lithium toxicity or serotonin syndrome.

38. **Answer: C.** Trifluoperazine

Trifluoperazine (Stelazine), thiothixene (Navane), haloperidol, and pimozide are high-potency antipsychotics.

39. **Answer: A.** Male sex

Women are more at risk than are men. Elderly people and patients with brain damage, mental retardation, and alcohol and substance use are also at increased risk. Diabetes has also been implicated as a risk factor.

40. **Answer: B.** Muscarinic

This is the classical presentation of cholinergic rebound associated with the abrupt cessation of clozapine.

41. **Answer: C.** Pindolol

Sympathomimetic effects of pindolol have a role in augmentation of antidepressant medications.

42. **Answer: B.** Rabbit syndrome

Rabbit syndrome presents as focal perioral tremor (choreoathetoid nature) that develops in patients taking dopamine antagonists.

43. **Answer: E.** All the above

SSRI-induced sexual dysfunction is usually treated by drugs that block serotonin or augment catecholamine especially dopamine. The antiserotonergic antidotes that can be used are cyproheptadine, buspirone, nefazodone, and mianserin. Amantadine has both dopaminergic and adrenergic activity.

44. **Answer: C.** Oligohydramnios

Lithium exposure can result in fetal and neonatal cardiac arrhythmias, hypoglycemia and nephrogenic diabetes insipidus, changes in thyroid function, polyhydramnios, and a "floppy infant syndrome" similar to infants exposed to benzodiazepine exposure.

45. **Answer: E.** All the above

Pharmacogenetics plays an important role in determining the pharmacologic response. Patient's tendency to respond to a specific class/group of antidepressants may be familial. Polymorphism in the gene expressing the hepatic enzyme *N*-acetyltransferase, which degrades phenelzine, appears to be inherited in a Mendelian fashion. Phenelzine is eliminated by acetylation. Slow versus rapid acetylation accounts for the toxic effect of phenelzine across individuals and different ethnic groups.

46. **Answer: C.** Fluoxetine

Fluoxetine has the half-life of 4 to 6 days, and its active metabolite norfluoxetine has a half-life of 4 to 16 days, which is the longest half-life of any of the SSRIs or their active metabolites. With its long elimination half-life, withdrawal symptoms do not occur with fluoxetine. Propranolol, clonidine, paroxetine, and venlafaxine are known to cause withdrawal symptoms.

47. **Answer: C.** *ß*-Adrenergic receptor antagonists

Psychotropics with high anticholinergic activity when combined with anticholinergic drugs such as benztropine can cause life-threatening anticholinergic intoxication syndrome. Dopamine antagonists, MAOIs, tricyclics, and tetracyclics have high anticholinergic activity. *ß*-Adrenergic receptor antagonists can be safely administered with benztropine.

48. **Answer: D.** Fluoxetine

Carbamazepine induces several hepatic enzymes resulting in lowering the plasma concentrations of the coadministered drugs. By inducing CYP3A4, it decreases levels of clozapine, lamotrigine, ethosuximide, and nefazodone. Clinical efficacy and plasma concentration of lamotrigine decrease to a clinically significant extent not only with carbamazepine but also with oxcarbazepine. Clozapine and carbamazepine should not be used concurrently because both have the potential to cause bone marrow suppression and may cause asterixis. Fluoxetine increases the level of carbamazepine because fluoxetine inhibits CYP3A.

49. **Answer: B.** SSRI-induced anorgasmia

SSRI-induced anorgasmia is treated with drugs that block serotonin or augment catecholamine especially dopamine. The antiserotonergic antidotes that can be used include cyproheptadine, buspirone, nefazodone, and mianserin. β-Adrenergic receptor antagonists have a role in the treatment of lithium-induced postural tremor, tricyclic-induced tremor, neuroleptic-induced akathisia, and aggressive behavior.

50. **Answer: D.** D_2 receptor supersensitivity

Clozapine has strong antagonistic properties at the receptors D_1 and D_4 and weak antagonism at D_2. It is highly anticholinergic and has 5-HT_2 antagonist effects. Clozapine does not cause D_2 receptor supersensitivity. Dopamine receptor supersensitivity refers to the phenomenon of increase in density of postsynaptic D_2 receptors. Conventional agents are known to cause supersensitivity.

51. **Answer: A.** Cyproheptadine

This patient has serotonin syndrome secondary to the use of multiple serotonergic drugs. Prompt initiation of cyproheptadine is recommended in the treatment of serotonin syndrome. Bromocriptine is contraindicated in this patient. Quetiapine, carbamazepine, and benztropine are not indicated in the treatment of serotonin syndrome.

52. **Answer: A.** Meprobamate

Meprobamate can be used to treat anxiety. In view of its additive sedating effects, abusive potential, and lethality in overdose, it is not used frequently. All other agents in the question stem do not have a role in the treatment of anxiety.

53. **Answer: D.** Cyproheptadine

Cyproheptadine causes weight gain and can be used in patients with anorexia nervosa.

54. Answer: D. Phenobarbital

Flumazenil does not reverse the effects of barbiturates or opioids. It is used for the reversal of zaleplon, zolpidem, and benzodiazepines overdose.

55. Answer: A. Alprazolam toxicity

Nefazodone inhibits oxidative metabolism mediated by CYP3A (metabolizes alprazolam), which could result in the increase of alprazolam level. It is recommended to reduce the dose of alprazolam to 50% while initiating nefazodone. Nefazodone rarely cause hepatotoxicity requiring liver transplant, and there are cases of death from its use. However, the patient described in the question stem does not present with symptoms of hepatotoxicity. Nefazodone concentration is not affected by alprazolam.

56. Answer: C. Amantadine

Rabbit syndrome presents as focal perioral tremor (choreoathetoid nature) that develops in patients taking dopamine antagonists. Amantadine is the preferred choice because this patient has closed-angle glaucoma and anticholinergics will worsen his medical conditions.

57. Answer: A. Triggering the influx of chloride into the cell and thus creating an inhibitory effect on neuronal cells

Barbiturate, benzodiazepine, and nonbenzodiazepine hypnotic drugs are positive allosteric modulators of the $GABA_A$-receptor complex. By binding to a distinct site on the receptor, these drugs trigger the influx of chloride into the cell and thus creating an inhibitory effect on neuronal cells.

58. **Answer: C.** Women with severe episodes but at moderate risk for relapse in the short term should be tapered before conception but reinstituted after 7 to 9 weeks

Cardiogenesis is complete around 9 to 11 weeks of gestation, and lithium should be restarted only in the second trimester. The risk for Ebstein anomaly after prenatal lithium exposure rises from 1 in 20,000 to 1 in 1,000, so women with mild and infrequent episodes of illness should be gradually (>2 weeks) tapered before conception. However, women with severe and frequent episodes of illness, lithium should be continued throughout the pregnancy in conjunction with counseling on teratogenicity.

59. **Answer: D.** Lithium

Risperidone when administered with clozapine may decrease the risperidone clearance. Concurrent use of clozapine and benztropine may result in increased anticholinergic side effects such as dry mouth and sedation. There is no DDI reported with quetiapine. Clozapine, lithium, and carbamazepine, when administered alone and when used concurrently with the either one of these agents, increase the risk of asterixis.

60. **Answer: A.** Suprachiasmatic nucleus

Ramelton is an agonist on MT$_1$ and MT$_2$ receptor. It has no affinity for GABA receptors. MT$_1$ and MT$_2$ receptor is located in suprachiasmatic nucleus, which regulates the sleep–wake cycle.

61. **Answer: D.** Cyproheptadine

Cyproheptadine acts both on histamine and serotonin receptors. Promethazine, diphenhydramine, and hydroxyzine are all antihistaminic agents. Benztropine is an anticholinergic agent.

62. **Answer: B.** Zolpidem

Zolpidem may be safer in pregnant women and is a category B medication in pregnancy. Lorazepam may cause floppy baby syndrome but less frequently than diazepam. A higher incidence of respiratory depression in newborn infants was reported with maternal lorazepam use. Zaleplon is a category C medicine in pregnancy.

63. Answer: D. Food significantly enhances the bioavailability of sodium oxybate

Food significantly decreases the bioavailability of sodium oxybate, and it is recommended to take the drug on empty stomach. It is indicated in the treatment of excessive daytime sleepiness and cataplexy in patients with narcolepsy. It is a schedule III drug under the Controlled Substances Act.

64. Answer: C. 1,200 mg per day

Neonatal risks may be reduced by being careful not to exceed the VPA dose of 1,000 mg per day or a serum concentration of 70 μg per ml.

65. Answer: B. The risk is higher with concomitant phenytoin therapy

Incidence of Steven–Johnson syndrome in adults is about 0.1%. Adding phenytoin does not increase the risk of lamotrigine-induced Steven–Johnson syndrome. The risk is higher if the dosage is escalated too rapidly, and in most cases, it appears after 2 to 8 weeks of therapy. Lamotrigine-induced Steven–Johnson syndrome is rarely associated with multiple organ failure.

66. Answer: A. It is a likely result of carbamazepine's antidiuretic effect

Carbamazepine-induced hyponatremia is likely a result of carbamazepine's antidiuretic effect. Old age and female gender are an independent risk factor for hyponatremia. Incidence varies from 1.8% to 40%.

67. Answer: E. All of the above

Absorptions of ziprasidone, diazepam, vilazodone, and carbamazepine are enhanced when taken with food.

68. **Answer: B.** VPA

VPA should be avoided as a first-line agent in any women of reproductive age.

69. **Answer: E.** All of the above

Electrocardiographic changes occur with thioridazine, pimozide, chlorpromazine, and ziprasidone.

70. **Answer: E.** All of the above

Clozapine when combined with captopril, sulfonamides, propylthiouracil, or carbamazepine increases the risk of bone marrow suppression and agranulocytosis because each agent on its own has this property. Carbamazepine may decrease the level of clozapine up to 60% when administered together.

71. **Answer: D.** Atypical agents produce depolarization blockade both in A_9 and A_{10} dopamine neurons

Fos protein is produced by neuroleptic agents' effects on the c-fos gene. Both conventional and atypical neuroleptics increase c-fos in nucleus accumbens resulting in improvements in positive symptoms. Atypical agents increase c-fos levels in the prefrontal cortex that correlates with the improvement in negative symptoms. Only conventional antipsychotic agents increase c-fos in striatum. Conventional agents produce depolarization blockade both in A_9 (substantia nigra) and A_{10} (mesolimbic) dopamine neurons and not the atypical agents.

72. **Answer: B.** Leukopenia

Carbamazepine is known to cause leukopenia, and lithium is associated with leukocytosis. Thus, it can mitigate carbamazepine-induced leukopenia. Lithium does not cause syndrome of inappropriate antidiuretic hormone but is associated with nephrogenic diabetes insipidus.

73. **Answer: C.** 40%

The incidence of SSRI-resistant OCD is 40%.

74. **Answer: A.** Inhibition of colony-stimulating factor in the bone marrow

Inhibition of colony-stimulating factor in the bone marrow is the most likely mechanism of neutropenia associated with carbamazepine therapy.

75. **Answer: B.** Zaleplon has a half-life of over 6 hours

Zaleplon has a rapid onset of action. It has an ultra short half-life of 1 hour. Zolpidem is a selective $GABA_A$ receptor α_1-subunit agonist used in the management of insomnia. The risk of dependence with zolpidem increases with the duration of treatment.

76. **Answer: D.** Unpleasant taste is a very common side effect

Eszopiclone (Lunesta) causes unpleasant taste, which is a very common side effect. It is not structurally related to zaleplon and is an S (+) enantiomer of racemic zopiclone. It is a category C drug and is not recommended during pregnancy or breast-feeding.

77. **Answer: C.** Mental status changes, hypertension, and myoclonus

Serotonin syndrome may occur as a result of a DDI between tramadol and paroxetine because both these agents inhibit serotonin reuptake. Tramadol is a weak μ-opioid analgesic and weak reuptake inhibitor of serotonin and norepinephrine. Serotonin syndrome commonly presents as changes in mental status, hyperthermia, autonomic hyperactivity, and neuromuscular abnormalities. Analgesic effect of tramadol may decrease when combined with paroxetine.

78. **Answer: C.** John Cade

Dr. John Cade, an Australian psychiatrist, discovered the mood stabilization effects of lithium bicarbonate. Leo Sternbach, a Polish chemist, synthesized about 40 derivatives from benzo-1,2,6-oxadiazepine, which were pharmacologically inert, and Lowell Randall later discovered chlordiazepoxide from the one, left over agent by Leo Sternbach. Arvid Carlsson, a Swedish scientist, discovered the neurotransmitter dopamine, and Emil Kraepelin, a German psychiatrist, coined the term *dementia praecox* and is considered to be the founder of modern psychiatry and psychopharmacology.

79. Answer: C. Sodium bicarbonate

Dysrhythmia induced by TCA should be treated with sodium bicarbonate. If sodium bicarbonate fails, then lidocaine is indicated. Ammonium chloride has no indication in the management of TCA-induced cardiac arrhythmia/dysrhythmia. Physostigmine reverses anticholinergic effects of TCA, but the risks often outweigh the benefits. Hence, it should only be used in patients with coma when other standard therapy fails.

80. Answer: E. All of the above

Clinical manifestations of tricyclic overdose are traditionally categorized as anticholinergic effects, cardiovascular effects, and central nervous effects. TCA toxicity is mediated by reuptake inhibition of norepinephrine, membrane-stabilizing effect on the myocardium, and antagonism at adrenergic and cholinergic receptors.

81. Answer: C. What the body does to the drug

Pharmacokinetics is defined as what the body does to the drug, whereas pharmacodynamics describes what the drug does to the body. Psychopharmacogenetics is the study of genetic differences in the behavioral response to pharmacologic agents. Pharmacokinetic variability refers to the genetic differences in the absorption and degradation of drugs, and pharmacodynamic variability is the genetic differences in tissue sensitivity to drugs.

82. Answer: B. Eosinophilia

Eosinophilia has been reported to occur with clozapine. An elevated eosinophil count may be an indicator of developing neutropenia. One may interrupt therapy when the eosinophil count >4,000 per mm^3, whereas one may resume therapy when the eosinophil count <3,000 per mm^3.

83. Answer: E. All of the above

Chronic SSRI use is reported to be associated with short-term memory impairment, concentration problems, and disturbances in sleep, particularly, decrease in Non-Rapid Eye Movement sleep (NREM) sleep and increase in wakefulness. Thus, chronic SSRI use is known to cause yawning, exhaustion, and fatigue.

84. **Answer: D.** CYP1A2

Fluvoxamine is a potent inhibitor of CYP1A2, and clozapine is a substrate of CYP1A2. Hence, fluvoxamine may decrease the metabolism of clozapine, resulting in increased serum concentrations. Thus, it is prudent to lower the dose of clozapine to avoid toxicity.

85. **Answer: E.** All of the above

Antipsychotic drugs cause weight gain through their effect on serotonin, histamine, dopamine, and adrenergic receptors. The CATIE trial, which included 1,493 participants from 57 US institutions, concluded that the greatest body weight gain was observed with olanzapine, whereas smaller increases were recorded after administration of risperidone or quetiapine.

86. **Answer: C.** History of liver cirrhosis

Bupropion is contraindicated in patients with a history of seizure disorder, febrile childhood seizures, head injury, CNS tumor, and eating disorder because it lowers their seizure threshold. It is safe in patients with history of liver cirrhosis. Bupropion has some evidence in treating patients with primary biliary cirrhosis.

87. **Answer: A.** Stop aripiprazole and start him on a different antipsychotic

Aripiprazole is primarily metabolized by CYP2D6 and CYP3A4. Rifampicin induces CYP2C9 and CYP3A4 enzymes, thereby decreasing the level and efficacy of aripiprazole in the blood. So aripiprazole should be switched to different antipsychotic.

88. **Answer: D.** Lamotrigine

Hyponatremia is associated with many psychotropic medications. The main cause is the SIADH. Drugs such as carbamazepine, oxcarbazepine, TCAs, SSRIs, and antipsychotics may cause hyponatremia. Lamotrigine is not associated with hyponatremia.

89. Answer: B. Haloperidol

The therapeutic index of a given drug is defined as the ratio of the toxic dose to its therapeutic dose. Lithium and nortriptyline both have a narrow therapeutic index. Haloperidol has wide therapeutic index.

90. Answer: B. Hemodialysis is indicated in overdose with venlafaxine

Venlafaxine overdose is managed with gastric lavage and supportive measures. Among patients with lithium overdose, hemodialysis should be initiated when serum level is >4.0 mEq per L or if the patient has serious signs and symptoms of lithium toxicity. Hemodialysis in VPA overdose patients improves the outcome. Low protein-binding drugs can be removed from the systemic circulation by hemodialysis as opposed to high protein-binding drugs.

91. Answer: A. Hyperkalemia

Haloperidol may be associated with the development of QTc prolongation and torsades de pointes. Hypokalemia is a risk factor for the development of torsades de pointes, but not hyperkalemia. The other risk factors are hypoxia, hypomagnesemia, hypocalcemia, liver failure, heart failure, and the use of class IA and III antiarrhythmics.

92. Answer: B. Mirtazapine

Mirtazapine has modest anticholinergic effects. The side effects experienced by the patient are probably because of the additive anticholinergic side effects of amitriptyline and mirtazapine.

93. Answer: D. Availability of transdermal preparation

Guanfacine is not available as transdermal preparation. It is less sedating than clonidine is, and it requires less frequent dosing. The withdrawal symptoms are less severe when compared with clonidine.

94. Answer: B. 0.05% to 0.1%

First trimester exposure to lithium results in 0.05% and 0.1% prevalence of Ebstein anomaly when compared with general population.

95. **Answer: B.** 4 hours

Venlafaxine's half-life is only 4 hours. Hence, even a single missed dose can cause withdrawal symptoms.

96. **Answer: B.** Protriptyline

Protriptyline, a secondary amine TCA, does not cause sedation. It has a role in the treatment of narcolepsy. All the TCA in the question stem causes sedation.

97. **Answer: D.** The drug is mainly metabolized by the CYP3A4 P450 isozyme

Duloxetine is an SNRI- and FDA-approved drug for the treatment of major depressive disorder, GAD, fibromyalgia, chronic musculoskeletal pain, and diabetic neuropathy. It is not approved for stress urinary incontinence, although it has some effect on urethral resistance. It is metabolized by CYP2D6 and CYP1A2.

98. **Answer: C.** No dietary restrictions are required when dosed at 6 mg per 24 hours

The action of selegiline is related to its irreversible inhibition of MAO, with greater affinity for type B (MAO-B), the major form of the enzyme in the human brain. Selegiline becomes a nonselective inhibitor of both MAO-A and MAO-B at doses of 9 mg per 24 hours and 12 mg per 24 hours transdermal patch, respectively. At these doses, tyramine-mediated hypertensive reactions from MAO-A blockade may occur. The most common side effect with the selegiline transdermal patch is application site reaction. The incidence of orthostatic hypotension in clinical trials is about 9.8%. Selegiline is only indicated for the treatment of major depression disorder and not approved for pediatric use.

99. **Answer: B.** Clomipramine

Clomipramine is FDA approved in the treatment of OCD. The drug blocks the reuptake of serotonin (5-HT) that is believed to contribute to its efficacy in OCD. Clomipramine can lower seizure threshold and hence should be avoided in patients with history of head injury and seizures. Although bupropion can also cause seizures, it does not have robust data supporting its efficacy in OCD.

100. **Answer: A.** Isotretinoin

Isotretinoin is a therapy for severe acne. In 1998, the US FDA issued a warning to physicians regarding a possible association with depression, psychosis, suicidal ideation, and suicide. The relationship between oral contraceptives, atenolol and varenicline, and drug-induced depression is inconclusive. The typical neuropsychiatric complication of digoxin therapy is delirium.

101. **Answer: B.** Nortriptyline

Among the TCAs, secondary amines such as nortriptyline, desipramine, and protriptyline are known to block the reuptake of norepinephrine and, to a lesser extent, serotonin.

102. **Answer: C.** Venlafaxine

Tamoxifen's effects in the breast depend on its ability to antagonize estrogen. Tamoxifen's antiestrogen affinity is thought to depend on the activity of its primary metabolite, endoxifen. Tamoxifen is metabolized to endoxifen through the liver enzyme CYP2D6. SSRIs (especially paroxetine, fluoxetine, bupropion, and duloxetine) are potent CYP2D6 inhibitors that can reduce the conversion of tamoxifen to endoxifen, thereby potentially reducing the efficacy of tamoxifen as a breast cancer therapy. Venlafaxine is a weak CYP2D6 inhibitor and hence is the preferred agent in the treatment of depression in women receiving tamoxifen.

103. **Answer: D.** Quetiapine is FDA approved for the treatment of acute bipolar depression

Quetiapine regular and extended-release tablets are indicated for the acute treatment of depressive episodes associated with bipolar disorder, type I and type II. Lamotrigine is FDA approved for maintenance therapy of bipolar I disorder. The National Institute of Mental Health (NIMH) funded STEP-BD was a long-term outpatient study designed to find out which treatments, or combinations of treatments, are most effective for treating bipolar disorder. The STEP-BD trial concluded that the addition of an antidepressant medication to adequate, optimally dosed mood-stabilizing medications does not improve recovery from bipolar depression any more than adding a placebo. Moreover, adding an antidepressant did not increase the risk of a switch to mania or hypomania. Finally, the study demonstrated that the addition of intensive psychotherapy to standard mood stabilizer treatment was associated with better symptomatic recovery.

104. **Answer: A.** 100 mg

In patients stabilized on low daily oral haloperidol doses (up to 10 mg per day), the recommended dose of haloperidol decanoate is 10 to 15 times the previous daily oral dose administered IM monthly or every 4 weeks. In cases where the patient is at high risk for relapse, a starting dose of 20 times the previous oral dose can be utilized.

105. **Answer: C.** Clonazepam

Clonazepam has the longest half-life among the high-potency benzodiazepines. Other high-potency benzodiazepines are lorazepam, alprazolam, and triazolam. Temazepam is a low-potency benzodiazepine with short half-life, whereas diazepam and chlordiazepoxide are low-potency benzodiazepines with long half-lives.

106. **Answer: C.** α-Adrenergic receptors

Some side effects of risperidone may be explained by antagonistic effects at histamine H_1 (somnolence) and α-adrenergic (orthostatic hypotension) receptors. Risperidone has negligible affinity for cholinergic-muscarinic, β-adrenergic, or 5-HT_3 receptors.

107. **Answer: C.** Opiate dependence

Bupropion inhibits reuptake of serotonin, dopamine, and norepinephrine that is responsible for the efficacy in major depressive disorder and attention deficit hyperactivity disorder. It has no role in opiate dependence. SSRI-induced sexual dysfunction is related to its inhibiting effect on adrenergic mechanism of orgasmic function and dopaminergic function of sexual desire. Bupropion by inhibiting dopamine reuptake can increase dopamine function and hence can increase sexual desire and function.

108. **Answer: C.** Carbamazepine extended release (Equetro)

The extended release formulation of carbamazepine (Equetro) is FDA indicated in the management of bipolar, manic, or mixed states. Other agents listed have limited to no data in the management of acute mania.

109. Answer: A. Most patients discontinue antidepressant after consulting with their physician

Treatment nonadherence is a concern with antidepressant. Most patients discontinue on own and seldom consult with physician. Psychiatrists can improve treatment adherence by engaging patient in a shared decision-making process and by considering various issues such as dosing schedule, side effects, and the risk factor for DDI and comorbid psychiatric conditions.

110. Answer: D. Codeine

Tramadol, morphine, and propoxyphene are contraindicated with MAOI because they can cause serotonin syndrome, hypertensive crisis, and CNS depression. Codeine has no DDI with MAOIs and is safe for use.

111. Answer: A. Nefazodone

In contrast to SSRI, nefazodone and venlafaxine have ascending dose–antidepressant response curves. This is an indicative of a greater efficacy at higher doses and the possibility of a more rapid antidepressant response.

112. Answer: D. Prochlorperazine

Neuroleptic-induced akathisia is the least well-understood EPS. Prochlorperazine can actually cause akathisia and hence cannot be used in the management. Other agents listed are useful, with preference given to benzodiazepines and β-blockers.

113. Answer: B. The dose for T_3 for thyroid augmentation is typically 25 to 50 μg per day

T_3 augmentation is a well-established augmentation strategy in depression. It has been studied more extensively in TCA nonresponders rather than SSRI nonresponders. Serum levels of T_3 do not reliably predict treatment responses, and an adequate trial is between 7 and 14 days. T_3 augmentation is contraindicated in cardiac conditions, angina, and endocrine problems.

114. **Answer: E.** Theophylline

Theophylline increases lithium clearance and can lower serum levels. All other drugs increase lithium levels and have potential for toxicity.

115. **Answer: A.** As a result of DDI

Hyperammonemic encephalopathy can develop in patients on Depakote who either have urea cycle disorder or are concurrently on topiramate. Management is discontinuation of both drugs.

116. **Answer: B.** Risk of pregnancy

Risperidone, D_2 blocker, can increase prolactin levels and amenorrhea and can mimic menopause. Patients may also have fertility problems. On discontinuation of risperidone and initiation of aripiprazole, which is a partial dopamine agonist, the prolactin levels normalize and the fertility can be restored. Patients resume menses and are at risk of pregnancy if they do not use contraception. All other options are certainly possible; however, conveying the risk of pregnancy to the patient assumes greater priority.

117. **Answer: C.** OROS technology does not facilitate reduced dosing frequency

OROS is an advanced drug delivery technology that uses osmotic pressure as the driving force to deliver pharmacotherapy. A drug delivered using OROS by virtue of its slow ascending plasma concentration profile may have lower abuse potential. OROS technology releases drugs into the blood stream over a 24-hour period, decreases peak and trough level fluctuations, and allows for once-a-day dosing. The abuse potential for drug using OROS technology is low.

118. **Answer: E.** All of the above

Each of the four generally recognized phases of the pharmacokinetic sequence (absorption, distribution, metabolism, and elimination) is affected by pregnancy. This has important implications for pharmacotherapy of psychiatric disorders in pregnancy.

119. **Answer: B.** Paroxetine

First-trimester exposure to paroxetine appears to be associated with a significant increase in the risk of cardiac malformation. Studies indicate an odds ratio of 1.6 (95% confidence interval, 1.1 to 1.9), suggesting a 60% higher chance of a cardiac abnormality. Women should be advised that there are risks of depression relapse with the discontinuation of treatment. The risks and benefits of treatment should be weighed carefully.

120. **Answer: D.** Mirtazapine

Mirtazapine is not a dual reuptake inhibitor antidepressant. Its antidepressant activity is related to its ability to enhance central noradrenergic and serotonergic activity through its antagonist activity at central pre-synaptic α_2-adrenergic inhibitory autoreceptors and heteroreceptors. Venlafaxine, duloxetine, milnacipran, and TCAs such as amitriptyline inhibit the reuptake of both 5-HT and norepinephrine (NE).

121. **Answer: C.** Ziprasidone

A QTc interval that is >500 milliseconds is a risk factor for developing torsade de pointes. A QTc interval that is <440 milliseconds is considered normal. Among the atypical antipsychotics, ziprasidone has the greatest risk for QTc prolongation. During placebo-controlled trials, the use of ziprasidone 160 mg per day increased the QTc interval by an average of 10 milliseconds compared with placebo. Ziprasidone should be avoided in patients with a history of QTc prolongation or on medications associated with QTc prolongation. Routine monitoring of ECG is not necessary unless there are risk factors. The other atypical antipsychotics listed are also known to increase QTc intervals.

122. **Answer: A.** Tranylcypromine

Tranylcypromine is an irreversible long-acting blockade of MAO (MAO-A and MAO-B). Structurally, it resembles amphetamines and may produce more CNS stimulation than other MAOIs. Linezolid is an antibiotic with activity against gram-positive organisms. In addition, linezolid is a reversible and nonselective inhibitor of MAO. Spontaneous reports of serotonergic syndrome have been reported when linezolid is concomitantly administered with serotonergic agents. Maprotiline is not an MAOI, rather a tetracyclic antidepressant.

123. **Answer: B.** 41%

The CATIE study, a multisite clinical study sponsored by the National Institute of Mental Health, assessed the efficacy and safety/tolerability of olanzapine, quetiapine, risperidone, and ziprasidone compared with the conventional antipsychotic perphenazine in 1,460 patients diagnosed with chronic schizophrenia. A considerable percentage of patients (about 40.9%) enrolled in the CATIE study had metabolic syndrome. In another analysis, when the CATIE patients were compared with the matched sample of the US National Health and Nutrition Examination Survey study, CATIE men and women were more likely to have metabolic syndrome.

124. **Answer: D.** Nonsteroidal anti-inflammatory drugs (NSAIDs)

Although not formally approved by the FDA for fibromyalgia, cyclobenzaprine is effective for this condition. NSAIDs have little or no evidence for use in this population. Milnacipran, pregabalin, and duloxetine are FDA approved in fibromyalgia.

125. **Answer: C.** The probability of relapse during continuation therapy increased as a function of the number of treatment trials required to achieve remission

In the STAR*D study, the probability of relapse during continuation therapy increased as a function of the number of treatment trials required to achieve remission. Switching to or adding CBT after a first unsuccessful attempt at treating depression with an antidepressant medication is generally as effective as switching to or adding another medication. If first treatment with one SSRI fails, about one in four people who choose to switch to another medication got better, regardless of whether the second medication was another SSRI or a medication of a different class. It took an average of 6 to 7 weeks of treatment for participants to achieve a remission of depressive symptoms.

126. **Answer: D.** ECG

Carbamazepine is useful in the management of bipolar disorder. Because the drug can cause hepatic and renal dysfunction and can also suppress thyroid function, baseline and periodic monitoring of these parameters are recommended. Although carbamazepine usage is more commonly associated with neurologic side effects, rarely it may cause potentially life-threatening side effects like agranulocytosis, aplastic anemia, thrombocytopenia, and leukopenia. Hence, a CBC is recommended before and during carbamazepine therapy. Although carbamazepine shares structural similarities with the TCAs, routine ECGs are not recommended.

127. **Answer: C.** 150 mg

Trazodone has dose-dependent pharmacologic actions. It antagonizes 5-HT$_2$A receptors that along with its α_1-adrenergic and H$_1$ histamine antagonist properties make it clinically useful as a hypnotic. At dose above 150 mg per day, trazodone blocks the SERT, which has antidepressant properties.

128. **Answer: B.** Leukocytosis

Hematologic side effects are not very common with lithium therapy. However, benign leukocytosis is sometimes observed. The presence of leukocytosis is not an indication for discontinuing lithium therapy. Routine CBCs are not recommended.

129. **Answer: A.** Prescribe risperidone at approximately half the usual starting dose

The polymorphic enzyme CYP2D6 is involved in the metabolism of many psychotropic drugs. CYP2D6 is involved in the metabolism of risperidone to the active metabolite 9-hydroxy-risperidone. When both alleles of the CYP2D6 gene are inactive, the patient is referred to as poor metabolizer. Poor metabolizers of CYP2D6 are at greater risk of developing adverse drug reactions at therapeutic doses. Hence, a lower dose of psychotropic drug (in this case risperdione) is recommended.

130. **Answer: E.** All of the above

Prazosin is the most lipid soluble α_1-adrenergic blocker, which has demonstrated efficacy and safety in the treatment of nightmares and insomnia seen in PTSD. It can cause hypotension and dizziness after taking the first dose (first-dose phenomenon). It should not be prescribed along with trazodone because of the increased risk of priapism.

131. **Answer: E.** Monitor TSH at baseline and annually

One of the major concerns with atypical antipsychotics usage is their metabolic side effects such as weight gain, hyperglycemia, and diabetes. ADA/APA consensus guidelines recommend monitoring fasting plasma glucose and lipid profile at baseline, 3 months, and annually. BMI should also be measured on a monthly basis for 3 months and quarterly thereafter. TSH is not monitored.

132. **Answer: C.** Aripiprazole

In 2004, US FDA issued a black box warning for all antidepressant medications to stating the increased risk of suicidal thoughts and behavior in children, adolescents, and young adults. Because aripiprazole is FDA approved for use as an adjunctive treatment to antidepressants for major depressive disorder, it carries the black box warning for suicide risk. Aripiprazole is not approved for use in pediatric patients with depression.

133. **Answer: C.** Continue the same dose of risperidone

Antipsychotic trials should be of sufficient duration to allow for maximum benefit. Usually, this can range from 4 to 6 weeks and in some cases 8 to 12 weeks. Prematurely, increasing the dose or switching to a different antipsychotic can pose risk of side effects and worsening of symptoms. ECT is reserved for cases that do not respond to an adequate trial of antipsychotic and/or augmentation.

134. **Answer: B.** Triazolam

Triazolam has a very short half-life (<4 hours). Although triazolam is indicated for insomnia, the drug is not used widely because of a high frequency of psychiatric side effects. Flurazepam and nitrazepam both have longer half-lives (>48 hours). Diazepam's half-life is about 36 hours. Temazepam and clonazepam have relatively longer half-lives as well (approximately 8 hours).

135. **Answer: E.** All of the above

There is evidence to support that patients treated with second-generation (or atypical) antipsychotics experience weight gain, hyperglycemia, and lipid dysregulation. The FDA issued a warning regarding antipsychotic drugs in the elderly because of an increase in the risk of stroke and death in elderly demented patients.

136. **Answer: A.** Alprazolam toxicity

The patient is most likely experiencing alprazolam toxicity because of a DDI between carbamazepine and alprazolam. Carbamazepine increases hepatic metabolism of alprazolam and decreases alprazolam blood concentrations. In clinical situations such as this, sudden discontinuation of a potent cytochrome enzyme inducer such as carbamazepine can cause increase alprazolam levels and trigger symptoms of benzodiazepine toxicity.

137. **Answer: B.** Pimozide

Pimozide is an antipsychotic drug of the diphenylbutylpiperidine class. It is highly selective blocker of dopamine D_2 receptors. Quetiapine, loxapine, thioridazine, and ziprasidone all antagonize D_2 receptors, however, not as strongly as pimozide.

138. **Answer: C.** Increased slow-wave sleep

Zolpidem is a short-acting hypnotic used in management of insomnia. It increases slow-wave sleep that may cause rare side effects such as sleepwalking and nocturnal eating.

139. **Answer: A.** Topiramate is a carbonic anhydrase inhibitor

Topiramate is an anticonvulsant that acts through blockage of voltage-dependent sodium channels. It also inhibits the enzyme carbonic anhydrase leading to metabolic acidosis. Topiramate has no evidence in the management of mania. It increases the risk of kidney stones when used with other carbonic anhydrase inhibitors. It is also useful for the prophylaxis of migraine headaches in adults.

140. **Answer: C.** Hydrochlorothiazide

Lithium clearance is exclusively cleared by the kidney. Diuretics such as thiazides increase reabsorption of lithium in the proximal convoluted tubule leading to increased lithium levels. Loop diuretics do not promote lithium reabsorption. Osmotic diuretics like mannitol increase lithium excretion. Atenolol and spironolactone do not affect lithium clearance.

141. **Answer: C.** Vascular system

MAOIs inhibit the metabolic breakdown of dietary amines. When foods containing tyramine are consumed hypertensive crisis can occur. This is called as the cheese-effect. If foods containing tryptophan are consumed hyperserotonemia (elevated serotonin levels) occur. The exact mechanism by which tyramine causes a hypertensive reaction is not well understood, but it is assumed that tyramine displaces norepinephrine from neuronal storage vesicles. Headaches also can be caused by increased levels of histamine during MAOI treatment. Symptoms of histamine headaches include hypotension, colic, excessive salivation, and lacrimation.

142. **Answer: B.** $5\text{-}HT_2C$ and H_1 histaminergic

Mirtazapine is a tetracyclic antidepressant with hypnotic, antiemetic, and appetite stimulant actions. It acts on various subclasses of 5-HT, α, and H_1 receptors. Among these subclasses, $5\text{-}HT_2C$ and H_1 are the receptors that mediate appetite suppression. Antagonism of these receptors can increase appetite and weight gain during mirtazapine therapy.

143. Answer: B. Drug-induced sleep attack

The patient's symptoms are most likely because of side effect from pramipexole. Pramipexole is a dopamine agonist that is prescribed for the treatment of Parkinson disease and restless leg syndrome. Among the adverse effects, sleep attack (6%) is one of the serious side effects. Narcolepsy is characterized by excessive daytime sleepiness, cataplexy, sleep paralysis, and hypnogogic hallucinations. Conversion disorder presents with various neurologic symptoms like numbness, paralysis, seizures, and blindness without any neurologic cause. The patient's symptoms are not suggestive of a panic attack.

144. Answer: C. Has low risk for abuse

Buspirone is usually dosed two to three times a day. Its elimination half-life is about 2 to 3 hours. Buspirone does not provide rapid relief from anxiety symptoms like benzodiazepines. It has a low risk for abuse. It does not have any role in augmenting antipsychotics drugs. Buspirone is FDA approved for the treatment of anxiety and can be used to treat depression and nicotine dependence.

145. Answer: E. All of the above

Amitriptyline has maximal anticholinergic property among the tricyclics, whereas desipramine has the least anticholinergic property. Doxepin has antihistamine properties in addition to its sleep-promoting effect. Nortriptyline has a curvilinear therapeutic window.

146. Answer: E. None of the above

NMS refers to the combination of hyperthermia, rigidity, and autonomic dysregulation that can occur as a serious complication of the use of antipsychotic drugs. Suggested risk factors for NMS include male sex, young age, previous NMS, agitation requiring restraints, dehydration, low serum iron, and prolonged use of high-potency neuroleptics.

147. **Answer: A.** Fluoxetine

SSRIs are recommended as first-line treatments for affective instability and impulse dyscontrol seen in BPD. Among the SSRIs, fluoxetine has studied the most. TCAs and MAOIs have been investigated as alternative treatments for BPD, but the risk of adverse effects and toxicity is a limitation to their use in clinical practice. Antipsychotics such as olanzapine have demonstrated efficacy in domains such as anger, hostility, and impulsivity.

148. **Answer: E.** Paroxetine

Currently, paroxetine and sertraline are considered as first-line medications in women who need to start antidepressant treatment during the postnatal period and wish to continue breast-feeding. Although both drugs are excreted in breast milk, weight of an adequate body of evidence and/or expert consensus suggests that these drugs pose minimal risk to the infant when used during breast-feeding.

149. **Answer: A.** Doxepin

Doxepin has potent antihistaminergic properties that make it a useful drug in managing pruritus. It is FDA approved for the treatment of pruritus and is frequently used in the management of urticaria.

150. **Answer: A.** Cluster headache

Lithium is very effective for the prophylaxis of cluster headache. The exact mechanism is not known though.

151. **Answer: E.** All of the above

The learned helplessness model, reward model, behavioral despair/forced swim paradigm, and genetic models are used in antidepressant screening testing.

152. **Answer: E.** All of the above

Mirtazapine is associated with side effects such as somnolence, fatigue, an increase in serum cholesterol and neutropenia, and weight gain.

153. **Answer: B.** Decrease in serum cholesterol

Significant increases in atherogenic lipids (total cholesterol, very-low-density lipoprotein, low-density lipoprotein, and triglycerides) have been noted following the carbamazepine use in pediatric patients. Carbamazepine is known to decrease serum T_3 and T_4, impair dexamethasone suppression test, be associated with false positive pregnancy tests, and possibly increase the risk of skin rash.

154. **Answer: A.** α_1-Subunit

Zolpidem is a selective $GABA_A$ receptor α_1-subunit agonist used in the management of insomnia.

155. **Answer: C.** Bupropion

SSRI-induced sexual dysfunction is related to its inhibiting effect on adrenergic mechanism of orgasmic and dopaminergic function of sexual desire, which often results in noncompliance. Dopaminergic drugs are known to augment sexual function. Bupropion by inhibiting dopamine reuptake can increase dopamine function and hence can increase sexual desire and function. Thus, it could reverse SSRI-induced sexual side effects. Venlafaxine and aripiprazole have no role in the treatment of SSRI-induced sexual side effects. Few open-label studies reported that mirtazapine has a role in the treatment of SSRI-induced sexual side effect, but the efficacy needs to be systematically studied.

156. **Answer: A.** Coadministration of acetazolamide

Topiramate is a carbonic anhydrase inhibitor, and hence, coadministration of acetazolamide, which is an inhibitor of carbonic anhydrase, increases the risk of renal calculi. Concurrent use of furosemide or lithium with topiramate is safe, and no DDI is reported. Coadministration of divalproex and topiramate may increase the risk of hyperammonemia and encephalopathy.

157. **Answer: C.** Quetiapine

Quetiapine in higher doses has been associated with cataract formation in beagle dogs. However, there is no definite association between cataract formation in human and quetiapine use. The manufacturer recommends eye examinations to detect cataracts at baseline and at 6-month intervals in patients treated with quetiapine. Risperidone, olanzapine, aripiprazole, and haloperidol are not associated with cataract formation. However, typical neuroleptics such as chlorpromazine and several other phenothiazine drugs are associated with cataract formation.

158. **Answer: C.** Bethanechol

Bethanechol chloride, a cholinergic agent, is structurally related to acetylcholine and acts on muscarinic receptors, not on nicotinic receptors. It is used to treat TCA-induced peripheral anticholinergic side effects. Carbachol, a cholinergic agonist, is primarily used in the treatment of glaucoma, and methacholine is used for diagnosing bronchial hyperactivity; both these agents do not have a role in the management of TCA-induced peripheral anticholinergic side effects. Benztropine is used for medication-induced movement disorder and not for TCA-induced peripheral anticholinergic side effects.

159. **Answer: C.** Venlafaxine

Hyperhidrosis has been associated with antidepressants such as venlafaxine, SSRIs, and tricyclics.

160. **Answer: A.** Benztropine

Among the agents that are used to treat antidepressant-induced sweating, benztropine has the most evidence. Sweat glands besides the apocrine sweat glands are innervated by cholinergic nerves. Thus, benztropine, an anticholinergic agent, is used in the treatment of hyperhidrosis. Cyproheptadine and clonidine have some evidence as well.

161. **Answer: C.** Thiothixene

Thiothixene is a typical antipsychotic medication of the thioxanthene class. Trifluoperazine, chlorpromazine, mesoridazine, and fluphenazine are phenothiazine class of neuroleptics.

162. **Answer: C.** CYP3A4

Clarithromycin is a CYP3A4 inhibitor, and aripiprazole is a substrate for CYP3A4. Hence, when aripiprazole is coadministered with clarithromycin, aripiprazole concentration will be increased. The recommendation is to reduce the aripiprazole dose to half of its normal dose. If the patient is also taking a CYP2D6 inhibitor together with CYP3A4 inhibitor, the recommendation is to reduce the aripiprazole dose further to one-quarter of the normal dose.

163. **Answer: E.** Granulocytopenia

Granulocytopenia is seen with clozapine therapy.

164. **Answer: B.** ANC reaches 1,000 per mm

When ANC reaches 1,000 per mm, clozapine therapy should be discontinued, and rechallenge is not permitted. The recommendation is to monitor WBC every day until WBC count >3,000 per mm^3 and ANC >1,500 per mm^3 and twice weekly until WBC count >3,500 per mm^3 and ANC >2,000 per mm^3. Once WBC count >3,500 per mm^3, monitor with weekly WBC and ANC.

165. **Answer: A.** Bupropion

Bupropion is an inhibitor of CYP2D6 isoenzyme. Fluvoxamine is an inhibitor of CYP2C19, CYP1A2, and CYP2C9 isoenzymes. Risperidone and desipramine are substrates of CYP2D6 isoenzyme. Desvenlafaxine does not have significant clinical interactions.

166. **Answer: E.** Fluoxetine

Fluoxetine strongly inhibits the CYP2D6 isoenzyme. Bupropion also inhibits CYP2D6 isoenzyme but not as strong as fluoxetine. Fluvoxamine is an inhibitor of CYP1A2, CYP2C9, and CYP2C19 isoenzymes. Risperidone and desipramine are substrates of CYP2D6 isoenzyme.

167. **Answer: A.** CYP3A4

CYP3A4 is more abundant in the gut wall as well as in the liver. They are located on microsomal membranes and oxidatively metabolize not only medications but also endogenous prostaglandins and fatty acids. Besides lithium, CYP enzymes metabolize all the psychotropics.

168. **Answer: A.** Inhibition of p-glycoprotein within the gut wall results in increased drug efficacy

P-glycoproteins mediate distribution and bioavailability of medications. P-glycoprotein is an ATP-dependent transporter and is present in the plasma membrane of enterocytes that lines the GI tract, lines the capillaries of the blood–brain barrier, and is also found in the cells lining renal tubules. P-glycoprotein transporter has substrates, inhibitors, and inducers. Inducers decrease the levels of p-glycoprotein substrates, and p-glycoprotein inhibitors increase the blood levels of p-glycoprotein substrates.

169. **Answer: E.** Asenapine

Asenapine is an antagonist at $5\text{-HT}_1\text{A}$ receptor. Ziprasidone, vilazodone, and buspirone are all $5\text{-HT}_1\text{A}$ agonist.

170. **Answer: D.** Flurazepam

Flurazepam is not safe to use in a patient with hepatic insufficiency.

171. **Answer: D.** Lithium is as effective as antipsychotics in bipolar disorder with comorbid psychotic symptoms

Comorbid substance abuse is a predictor of poor response to lithium. It is not well tolerated in the elderly population. Lithium levels should be kept as low as 0.4 to 0.8 mEq per L in elderly because they are more sensitive to neurologic side effects even at lower lithium levels. Delirium can occur with serum levels of 1.5 mEq per L because of lithium's anticholinergic activity. Lithium is not as effective as anticonvulsants in the treatment of rapid cycling bipolar disorder. Lithium therapy is not recommended in patients with history of poor compliance.

172. **Answer: A.** Thrombocytopenia

Coadministration of clozapine and buspirone increases the risk of GI tract bleeding and hyperglycemia. When coadministered, treating physician should monitor for blood glucose levels, hematocrit, and signs and symptoms of GI tract bleeding.

173. **Answer: A.** Topiramate

Topiramate is a carbonic anhydrase inhibitor and hence increases the risk of renal calculi.

174. **Answer: D.** Presystemic elimination

First-pass effect is a phenomenon of presystemic elimination of the drug resulting in reduced concentration.

175. **Answer: C.** VPA

VPA poses the greatest risk of neural tube defects, and it is not recommended in women of childbearing age. Phenytoin, VPA, and carbamazepine are all class D drugs in pregnancy. Levetiracetam and lamotrigine are class C drugs in pregnancy.

176. **Answer: B.** Hemodialysis

Lithium toxicity is managed by fluid therapy to enhance lithium clearance. However, when the levels are high, that is, >2.5 mEq per L and in patients who are at risk for volume overload, that is, CHF, hemodialysis is indicated. Lithium is readily dialyzed because of water solubility, low volume of distribution, and lack of protein binding.

177. **Answer: C.** Postural hypotension

Sexual dysfunction, abdominal discomfort, asthenia, and weight gain are common side effects, but postural hypotension is the most common side effect of MAOI therapy.

178. **Answer: E.** All of the above

Clozapine is associated with QTc prolongation, myocarditis, cardiomyopathy, and pericarditis.

179. **Answer: C.** Topiramate

Topiramate has been most strongly associated with cognitive side effects.

180. **Answer: D.** Molindone

Molindone causes weight loss, and chlorpromazine causes weight gain. Among the atypical antipsychotics, olanzapine causes the most weight gain. The CATIE trial, which included 1,493 participants from 57 US institutions, concluded that the greatest body weight gain was observed with olanzapine, whereas smaller increases were recorded after administration of risperidone or quetiapine. A minor body weight decrease was observed with ziprasidone.

181. **Answer: C.** Clozapine is schedule II drug

Schedule II drugs are considered to have a strong potential for abuse or addiction but are indicated for legitimate medical use. Some examples of schedule II drug are narcotics such as morphine, oxycodone, and methadone. Clozapine is not a schedule II drug.

182. **Answer: B.** 40 mg per day

The recommended dose of IM ziprasidone is 10 to 20 mg. The maximum recommended daily dose of IM ziprasidone is up to 40 mg per day.

183. **Answer: B.** 15 to 30 minutes

Peak plasma concentrations of IM olanzapine are typically reached in 15 to 30 minutes, whereas oral dose takes about 4 hours.

184. **Answer: E.** Failure to respond to a trial of long-acting injectable antipsychotic agent

Kane et al. proposed criteria for treatment refractory schizophrenia based on cross-sectional, prospective, and previous treatment history. BPRS score >45, Clinical Global Impressions Scale (CGI) score >4, no episodes of good functioning in the previous 5 years, and failure to respond to at least three antipsychotic trials from two different chemical class of adequate duration dose such as 1,000 mg per day of chlorpromazine for 6 weeks, without significant symptom relief, or intolerance to a 6-week prospective trial of haloperidol at 10 to 60 mg per day.

185. **Answer: D.** 60 mg per day

Fluoxetine has shown to be effective in reducing binge eating and purging in bulimic women. The recommended dose of fluoxetine for bulimia nervosa is 60 mg per day on day 1. It is tolerated well, and perhaps fluoxetine is the only medication approved by FDA for bulimia.

186. **Answer: A.** In case of interruption of lamotrigine therapy for 7 days, it requires prior initial start-up dose and gradual retitration

Immune tolerance to lamotrigine is lost after interruption of dosage for >1 week, and hence, it requires prior initial start-up dose and gradual retitration.

187. **Answer: E.** All of the above

Dilated cardiomyopathy, myocarditis, heart failure, and sudden cardiac death are rare but recognized side effects of clozapine therapy.

188. **Answer: B.** Prescribe multiple but low doses of psychotropic medications

Prescribing multiple but low doses of psychotropic medications is not recommended in managing any psychiatric illness. BPD patients often require higher doses of SSRIs.

189. **Answer: A.** Bupropion

Bupropion is contraindicated in patients with seizure disorder. Paroxetine, venlafaxine, and mirtazapine are also known to decrease the seizure threshold and should be used with caution in a patient with history of seizures.

190. **Answer: A.** Increase in bioavailability

Ziprasidone's bioavailability increases by 2-fold when administered with food.

191. **Answer: E.** None of the above

Olanzapine, mirtazapine, clozapine, and carbamazapine have all been reported to decrease WBC counts.

192. **Answer: B.** Modafinil is a racemic compound, whose enantiomers have different pharmacokinetics

Modafinil is indicated for narcolepsy, obstructive sleep apnea, and shift work sleep disorder. Modafinil has reinforcing properties at higher dose. It is a racemic compound, and no differences between the enantiomers are reported in animal models. No data are available on humans yet. Modafinil is listed in schedule IV of the Controlled Substances Act. Headache is a common side effect with modafinil therapy.

193. **Answer: A.** The incidence of sustained hypertension with venlafaxine is dose dependent

Sustained increase in supine diastolic BP is dose dependent. The increase in BP with immediate-release venlafaxine is 3% for doses <100 mg per day, and BP increases up to 13% for doses >300 mg per day. The BP elevation is not transient.

194. **Answer: D.** Baclofen

Baclofen is an agonist at $GABA_B$ receptor. Diazepam is a benzodiazepine. Zolpidem exerts its sedative property by binding to the benzodiazepine receptor subunit of the $GABA_A$ receptor complex. Eszopiclone may binds allosterically at the GABA receptor complex domain and acts as a sedative agent.

195. **Answer: B.** Lithium

Lithium has data in upregulating neurotrophins including BDNF, nerve growth factor, and NT3 and acts as a neuroprotective agent.

196. **Answer: B.** Pramipexole

Pramipexole is a nonergot dopamine agonist that is indicated in the treatment of restless leg syndrome and Parkinson disease. There is growing evidence that it is useful in the treatment of depression.

197. **Answer: A.** Nortriptyline

Nortriptyline has the greatest evidence in the treatment of depression associated with Parkinson disease.

198. **Answer: D.** Olanzapine

Olanzapine has demonstrated efficacy in the treatment of acute and delayed chemotherapy-induced nausea and vomiting in patients receiving emetogenic chemotherapy. Mirtazapine is being studied, and there are some data suggesting its efficacy. Other agents listed do not have any role in the treatment of chemotherapy-induced nausea and vomiting.

199. **Answer: E.** None of the above

Selegiline is used in the treatment of Parkinson disease and depression. It is an MAO-B inhibitor that becomes MAO-A inhibitor at higher doses. SSRIs are contraindicated, and weight loss is reported in 5% of patients on selegiline therapy.

200. **Answer: E.** All of the above

Phenelzine when combined with amphetamine, methyldopa, methylphenidate, or buspirone may result in hypertensive crisis.

201. **Answer: A.** Nefazodone

Nefazodone has a black box warning for hepatotoxicity. It is associated with severe hepatotoxicity, sometimes requiring liver transplant. Desvenlafaxine, desipramine, paroxetine, and tranylcypromine are not associated with fatal hepatic failure.

202. **Answer: A.** Venlafaxine

Venlafaxine treatment has shown to be efficacious in decreasing hot flash. Clonidine is also used to treat hot sweats, but studies concluded that oral venlafaxine reduced the frequency of hot flash to a greater extent compared with clonidine.

203. **Answer: A.** It is associated with high prevalence of thyroid autoantibodies

Lithium-induced thyroiditis and thyroid dysfunction is thought to be mediated by an autoimmune response. Lithium may also worsen an underlying autoimmune thyroiditis by shifting the T-lymphocyte subpopulations.

204. **Answer: C.** Nortriptyline

Nortriptyline when administered with clonidine may result in hypertension because the combination decreases the antihypertensive effect of clonidine. No DDI of clonidine has been reported with paroxetine, fluoxetine, and bupropion. Mirtazapine when combined with clonidine may decrease the antihypertensive effect of clonidine.

205. **Answer: A.** CYP2D6 and CYP2C19

FDA approved the pharmacogenetic test using DNA array technology for genotyping CYP isoenzymes genes. The AmpliChip CYP450 test (Roche Molecular Systems) detected up to 33 CYP2D6 alleles and 3 CYP2C19 alleles. This test assists the clinician in determining the treatment formulation and optimal dosing of the medications that are metabolized by the CYP2D6 or CYP2C19.

206. **Answer: D.** Lithium inhibits vasopressin-stimulated cyclic AMP (cAMP) production, which is one of the primary factors contributing to the impaired urine concentrating ability

Lithium impairs kidneys' ability to concentrate the urine by inhibiting the activation of vasopressin-sensitive adenylate cyclase in renal epithelial cells and thus inhibiting cAMP production. The renal effects are reversible and related to the dose of lithium. Lithium-induced polyuria is highly prevalent, and it is estimated to be around 20% to 70%. It is often seen in prolonged treatment with lithium.

207. **Answer: A.** NMS

Dantrolene is indicated in the treatment of malignant hyperthermia and chronic spasticity. It is also frequently used in the treatment of NMS.

208. **Answer: E.** All of the above

VPA increases the concentration of 10 to 11 epoxide metabolites of carbamazepine causing carbamazapine toxicity. VPA clearance is increased when combined with carbamazepine, and hence, increased VPA dose may be required. Toxicity may emerge even at therapeutic serum CBZ levels. Carbamazepine toxicity manifests symptoms include ataxia, nystagmus, headache, vomiting, and seizures.

209. **Answer: B.** Clozapine

Clozapine reduces the risk of suicide by 75% to 80% in schizophrenic patients. The International Suicide Prevention Trial, a prospective study, investigated the effect of clozapine versus olanzapine and suicidal rates of patients with schizophrenia. It was concluded that clozapine is effective in reducing the risk of current suicidal behavior in patients with schizophrenia or schizoaffective disorder and in decreasing the number of suicide attempts in patients who are at high risk for suicide.

210. **Answer: D.** VPA-induced hepatic dysfunction resolves completely after discontinuing the drug

Children younger than 2 years are at increased risk for VPA induced hepatotoxicity, and the risk is higher if they are taking multiple anti-convulsants and have comorbid conditions such as mental retardation and organic brain disease. The risk is usually higher in the first 6 months of initiating the treatment. In some patients, hepatic dysfunction has progressed even after discontinuing VPA. The mechanism of hepatotoxicity is believed that VPA induces carnitine deficiency in young children that causes hepatotoxicity. Thus, carnitine supplementation may help in preventing the onset of hepatotoxicity.

211. **Answer: A.** Alprazolam

The therapeutic index of a given drug is defined as the ratio of the toxic dose to its therapeutic dose. Lithium, amitriptyline, clozapine, and carbamazepine have a narrow therapeutic index. Alprazolam and benzodiazepines in general have wide therapeutic index.

212. **Answer: B.** Thioridazine

Thioridazine is known to cause retinal pigmentation and visual impairment. Thioridazine-induced pigmentary retinopathy is dose related. Usually, it develops within 2 to 8 weeks after initiation of the treatment; even after thioridazine is discontinued, pigmentary changes may progress, but visual impairment usually improves.

213. **Answer: B.** Clozapine

Clozapine is useful in treatment refractory schizophrenia. Meltzer et al. have examined this further and concluded that about 30% of patients would respond by 6 weeks, a further 20% by 3 months, and an additional 10% to 20% by 6 months. Hence, it is encouraged to try clozapine therapy for at least 6 months before labeling the patient as resistant to clozapine.

214. **Answer: C.** Lithium

Literature supports that lithium therapy is associated with a lower suicide rate in patients with bipolar disorder.

215. **Answer: B.** Imipramine

Desipramine is the main metabolite of imipramine. Imipramine is a strong inhibitor of serotonin reuptake, but its metabolite desipramine is highly noradrenergic reuptake inhibitor.

216. **Answer: E.** All of the above

Pergolide, ropinirole, bromocriptine, and pramipexole are all dopamine receptor agonists.

217. **Answer: C.** Paroxetine

Paroxetine does not have any evidence in the treatment of neuropathic pain.

218. **Answer: B.** Risperidone

Risperidone is FDA approved for the treatment of irritability associated with autistic disorder.

219. **Answer: C.** The maximum dose should not exceed 50 mg every 2 weeks

Risperidone microspheres start releasing significant amount of drug, 3 weeks after the injection. Hence, supplementation with oral antipsychotic must continue for the first 3 weeks of therapy. When dose adjustment is made, clinical effects are expected after 3 weeks following the injection at higher dose. Steady plasma concentrations are achieved after the fourth injection, and therefore, dose adjustments cannot be made every 2 weeks.

220. **Answer: B.** Clomipramine

Clomipramine is the most serotonergic agent among the TCAs.

221. **Answer: A.** Carbamazepine

Carbamazepine is contraindicated in patients with a history of allergy to TCAs because it is structurally similar to imipramine.

222. **Answer: A.** Anticholinergic medications can decrease TD movements

TD is a delayed-onset abnormal involuntary movement after neuroleptic exposure. Recognition of TD should be followed by immediate tapering of the antipsychotic medication. Clonazepam has shown to be useful in TD. Clozapine can decrease TD movements, and botulinum toxin is not used in the treatment for TD. Anticholinergic medications are used in the management of extrapyramidal side effects, but they may worsen TD movements by increasing the supersensitivity of dopamine receptors. Hence, the recommendation is to stop the anticholinergic medications.

223. **Answer: C.** Full agonist at 5-HT$_2$A

Aripiprazole is a novel antipsychotic agent with partial agonistic action on D$_2$ and 5-HT$_1$A receptors and is an antagonist at 5-HT$_2$A receptors. It is a dopamine–serotonin system stabilizer.

224. **Answer: B.** Discontinue trazodone because it may precipitate symptoms of hypertension, hyperthermia, and mental status changes

Initiation of linezolid in this patient may result in serotonin syndrome. There is no DDI reported between linezolid with either ziprasidone or clonidine.

225. **Answer: C.** Binds less extensively to plasma proteins

Fluvoxamine is an FDA category C drug to be used in pregnancy. It is an inhibitor of CYP2C19, CYP1A2, and CYP2C9 isoenzymes. Fluvoxamine is metabolized by liver.

226. **Answer: E.** All of the above

Management of clozapine-induced hypersalivation can be challenging. Strategies such as reducing clozapine dose and chewing gum to promote swallowing are useful adjuncts to pharmacological interventions. Anticholinergic agent or α_2-agonist is frequently used to manage clozapine-induced hypersalivation.

227. **Answer: B.** Diazepam

Among the benzodiazepines, diazepam is the most lipophilic, and thus, it crosses the blood–brain barrier rapidly. This may account for its reinforcing properties and therefore it is likely to be abused. Alprazolam and lorazepam are less lipophilic compared with diazepam; however, they are high-potency benzodiazepines and associated with potential for abuse.

228. **Answer: B.** Baseline, 4 weeks, 8 weeks, 12 weeks, and quarterly

Current recommendation by the ADA/APA consensus management guidelines for monitoring BMI for patients receiving atypical antipsychotics is at baseline, 4 weeks, 8 weeks, 12 weeks, and quarterly.

229. **Answer: B.** Prophylactic anticholinergic medications

Anticholinergic medications are used in the management of extrapyramidal side effects, but they may worsen TD movements by increasing the supersensitivity of dopamine receptors. Hence, the recommendation is to stop the anticholinergic medications. Using anticholinergic medications is reported to increase the risk of developing TD.

230. **Answer: A.** Maculopapular rash

Many dermatologic reactions associated with lamotrigine use develop between 5 days and 8 weeks after starting lamotrigine. Many reactions are benign and are exanthematous, maculopapular, or morbilliform eruption with or without itching.

231. **Answer: E.** None of the above

VPA use is associated with adverse effects such as hair loss (5% to 10%), polycystic ovary syndrome (PCOS), hemorrhagic pancreatitis, and thrombocytopenia.

232. **Answer: C.** The greatest risk of rash with lamotrigine is during the first 2 weeks of treatment

Majority of the dermatologic reactions associated with lamotrigine use develop between 5 days and 8 weeks after starting lamotrigine.

233. **Answer: D.** They are found predominantly in gut and brain

CYP enzymes are found in gut and brain but predominantly in the liver. They are located on microsomal membranes and oxidatively metabolize not only medications but also endogenous prostaglandins and fatty acids. Besides lithium, CYP enzymes metabolize all the psychotropics.

234. **Answer: A.** Desipramine

Desipramine is a norepinephrine reuptake inhibitor. Doxepin is a TCA with significant antihistaminergic activity. Clomipramine is most serotonergic agent among TCAs. Desipramine and nortriptyline when compared with other tricyclics have lower anticholinergic adverse effects.

235. **Answer: B.** Polyuria

Lithium-induced polyuria is highly prevalent, and it is estimated to be around 20% to 70%. It is often seen with prolonged treatment with lithium.

236. **Answer: C.** Cyclobenzaprine

Coadministration of cyclobenzaprine and fluoxetine may result in an increased risk of QTc prolongation. Given her past medical history (PMH) of long QT syndrome, cyclobenzaprine is not recommended in this patient. Acetaminophen, baclofen, ibuprofen, and oxycodone may be safely used in a patient taking fluoxetine.

237. **Answer: C.** Shortened REM latency

Benzodiazepine prolongs the REM latency and increases K spindles in stage II. It decreases REM sleep and stage III and IV sleep.

238. **Answer: D.** Phenelzine

This patient meets criteria for MDD with atypical features. Traditionally, MAOIs are the treatment of choice. Meta-analysis reports that SSRIs are not as effective as MAOIs, and a small study reports duloxetine was effective in achieving response in 50% of the participants and 35% remitted. However, placebo-controlled studies are required to demonstrate efficacy of duloxetine in treating atypical depression.

239. **Answer: B.** It has no risk for addiction

Chloral hydrate is a nonbarbiturate hypnotic drug. It has FDA approval for insomnia, alcohol withdrawal syndrome and sedation, and it is as an adjunct analgesic in preoperative care and postoperative pain. It causes tolerance and dependence. Concurrent use with warfarin may increase the risk of bleeding.

240. **Answer: E.** All of the above

VPA may be a better choice in bipolar patients presenting with mixed episodes, rapid cycling, comorbid substance abuse, and increased impulsivity.

241. **Answer: C.** Can be used in the treatment of benzodiazepine withdrawal syndrome

Disadvantages of short half-life benzodiazepines are frequent dosing, withdrawal symptoms on abrupt discontinuation, anterograde amnesia, and rebound insomnia and anxiety. Long-acting benzodiazepines are used to treat benzodiazepine withdrawal syndrome.

242. **Answer: B.** Metoclopramide

Dopaminergic drugs are associated with three types of dyskinesia such as dyskinetic movements secondary to the use of levodopa, withdrawal dyskinetic movements that could be reversible, and irreversible TD. Metoclopramide is known to induce withdrawal dyskinetic movements on sudden discontinuation after chronic therapy. None of the other agents in the question stem cause withdrawal dyskinetic movements.

243. **Answer: D.** Absence of CPK elevations rules out a diagnosis of NMS

NMS is a life-threatening emergency associated with neuroleptic use. CPK elevation in NMS may vary between 1,000 IU per L and as high as 100,000 IU per L. Mild to moderate CPK elevation is not specific for NMS. Significant CPK elevations can occur with IM injections, physical restraints, and agitation. CPK elevation >1,000 IU per L is more specific for NMS. Absence of CPK elevations does not rule out a diagnosis of NMS.

244. **Answer: E.** All of the above

Concurrent use of selegiline with carbamazepine or oxcarbamazapine may result in an increase in selegiline plasma concentrations. When selegiline is combined with dextroamphetamine or methylphenidate, it may result in hypertensive crisis.

245. **Answer: C.** Sertraline

Cyclobenzaprine should be avoided in a patient taking duloxetine because this combination may increase the risk of serotonin syndrome. MAOIs are contraindicated and avoided in a patient on cyclobenzaprine. It may result in hypertensive crises or seizures. When cyclobenzaprine is combined with fluoxetine, it may increase the risk of QTc prolongation. Sertraline has no DDI with cyclobenzaprine and is safe to coadminister.

246. **Answer: B.** Olanzapine extended release injectable suspension

PDSS is reported with olanzapine extended release injectable suspension.

247. **Answer: B.** Prazosin

Prazosin, commonly used in the treatment of nightmares associated with PTSD, is most notorious for producing a first-dose phenomenon. It may cause idiosyncratic hypotensive response, which is very rare but serious. To avoid this, prazosin is scheduled as 1 mg at bedtime for three consecutive nights and subsequent titration to 10 mg or more until nightmares are controlled and sleep is restored.

248. **Answer: B.** Venlafaxine

The patient described in the vignette has treatment-resistant depression. He has failed two SSRIs, and it would be reasonable to consider an SNRI such as venlafaxine. Concurrent use of mirtazapine or nortriptyline in a patient taking clonidine may result in decreased antihypertensive effects. rTMS is indicated in a patient who failed one antidepressant treatment, and more data are needed to validate its efficacy in treatment-resistant depression.

249. **Answer: B.** SJW is a potent inhibitor of CYP3A4

Concurrent use of SSRIs and SJW may result in an increased risk of serotonin syndrome. SJW is a CYP3A4 inducer and not an inhibitor. SJW use is associated with diminished clinical effectiveness or increased dosage requirements for all CYP3A4 substrates. Cyclosporine efficacy is reduced when coadministered with SJW, and SJW is not recommended in organ transplant patients.

250. **Answer: D.** Mirtazapine

Mirtazapine is a potent 5-HT$_3$ blocker and thus acts as an antinausea agent.

251. **Answer: B.** Lithium tremors tend to be slow and rhythmic

Lithium tremors tend to be coarse and present at rest. Lithium tremors are made worse by movement. Studies report a wide range of incidence of lithium tremor between 4% and 65%. Management of lithium tremors include changing the dose or preparation of lithium, decreasing or discontinuing other medications that might cause tremors, and treating with ß-blockers such as metoprolol. Severe tremor may be a manifestation of lithium toxicity and should be evaluated and managed appropriately.

252. **Answer: B.** Flurazepam

Triazolam has a very short half-life (<4 hours). Flurazepam and nitrazepam both have longer half-lives (>48 hours), but flurazepam has the longest half-life of 40 to 250 hours. Diazepam's half-life is about 36 hours. Temazepam has a half-life of about 8 hours.

253. **Answer: A.** The existence of a curvilinear therapeutic window

The primary reason for monitoring plasma nortriptyline concentrations during the treatment of major depression is for the existence of a nortriptyline curvilinear therapeutic window.

254. **Answer: C.** 65% to 70%

PET studies indicate that 65% to 70% of D_2 receptor occupancy correlates with maximal antipsychotic efficacy.

255. **Answer: B.** Activated charcoal is helpful

Gastric decontamination should be the first-line management of tricyclic overdose after supportive measures. Activated charcoal can be administered up to 12 hours because TCA slows the gastric emptying. Dialysis has no role in the management of tricyclic overdose. Dysrhythmia induced by TCA should be treated with sodium bicarbonate. If sodium bicarbonate fails, then lidocaine is indicated. Ammonium chloride has no indication in the management of TCA overdose.

256. Answer: E. All of the above

Higher neonatal lithium concentrations are associated with significantly lower Apgar scores and higher CNS and neuromuscular complications. Stopping lithium 1 to 2 days before the delivery is likely to improve the neonatal outcomes.

257. Answer: E. None of the above

Sexual side effects in women on trazodone therapy are priapism of the clitoris, spontaneous orgasm, and increase or decrease in libido.

258. Answer: C. Molindone

Molindone has the lowest propensity to lower the seizure threshold. Among the typical antipsychotics, chlorpromazine has the greatest risk, and among the second-generation antipsychotics, clozapine has the greatest risk of inducing seizures.

259. Answer: B. 20% to 30%

Estimated mortality rate with NMS is about 20% to 30%.

260. Answer: E. None of the above

Asenapine is FDA approved for the management of acute mixed or manic episodes of bipolar I disorder and acute treatment of schizophrenia. It is well tolerated, has neutral metabolic effects, has minimal effects on prolactin, and has lower extrapyramidal side effects.

261. Answer: A. Steady-state lithium levels are attained after 2 days of constant dosing

Steady-state lithium levels are attained after 5 days of a dose adjustment, and hence, it is recommended to check the lithium level 5 days after initiating lithium or after a dose change. Serum lithium levels 12 hours post dose are 30% higher in patients taking the SR preparation compared with the IR preparation. Elderly patients require more frequent monitoring of serum lithium levels because of several reasons—their lithium levels fluctuate even without any dose adjustments and they are also more susceptible to lithium toxicity at low serum levels. There are commercially available tests kits that provide convenient and accurate measure of blood lithium levels in the office setting.

262. **Answer: E.** None of the above

Fetal echocardiogram is recommended between 16 and 18 weeks of gestation. Caution should be exercised regarding maternal NSAID use because of the DDI with lithium. Withholding lithium therapy for 24 to 48 hours because of delivery is shown to improve neonatal outcomes.

263. **Answer: E.** All of the above

PDSS results from probable accidental intravascular injection of olanzapine long-acting preparation. Current management is to treat symptomatically and supportive measures. Symptoms of PDSS are sedation or delirium related, such as motor impairment, cognitive impairment, disorientation, confusion, ataxia, change in level of consciousness, and dysarthria. Other symptoms are general malaise, agitation, aggression, and hypertension.

264. **Answer: E.** All of the above

Ziprasidone could be life threatening when administered to the patients with QTc >500 milliseconds and with a history of recent MI, or when a patient is in heart failure or arrhythmia.

265. **Answer: D.** It resolves spontaneously despite continued treatment

Leukopenia associated with carbamazapine therapy does not predispose patients to infections, and it is not a strong indicator of development of agranulocytosis. Incidence of carbamazepine-induced leukopenia is 2.1%. It resolves spontaneously despite continued treatment.

266. **Answer: B.** Hypotension

Orthostatic hypotension is a frequent side effect during MAOI therapy. There is some evidence that the orthostatic hypotension may resolve after 4 weeks of therapy, which is not the case with TCAs. BP monitoring is recommended at 3 to 4 weeks after medication is initiated. If a patient develops hypotension on MAOI therapy, dose changes should be gradual.

267. **Answer: E.** None of the above

Carbamazepine, lamotrigine, phenobarbital, and VPA are all associated with Stevens–Johnson syndrome. It is an exfoliative, autoimmune disorder of the skin and the mucous membranes caused by adverse drug reaction.

268. **Answer: B.** The drug's active metabolite threohydrobupropion is primarily responsible for the occurrence of seizures

Threohydrobupropion is less potent than bupropion, hence not responsible for the occurrence of seizures.

269. **Answer: C.** Fluvoxamine

Coadministration of fluvoxamine in a patient taking olanzapine may result in an increased risk of adverse effects from olanzapine. There is no DDI when paroxetine, fluoxetine, or buspirone is administered with olanzapine.

270. **Answer: C.** Temazepam

Alprazolam, clonazepam, lorazepam, and triazolam are high-potency benzodiazepines, whereas temazepam is a low-potency benzodiazepine. Other low-potency benzodiazepines are oxazepam, chlordiazepoxide, clorazepate, diazepam, and flurazepam.

271. **Answer: A.** SJW

SJW is contraindicated in a patient on selegiline. Concurrent use of these two agents may result in an increased risk of serotonin syndrome and hypertensive crisis.

272. **Answer: B.** Pronounced sedation on low-dose mirtazapine therapy rather than high-dose mirtazapine therapy

Mirtazapine preferentially blocks the histamine-1 receptor at low doses, resulting in profound sedation at low doses. At higher doses, mirtazapine blocks the α_2-adrenergic receptor.

273. **Answer: C.** Hematopoietic system

Concurrent use of lithium and carbamazepine may result in additive side effects on CNS. Neurotoxicity may manifest in the form of weakness, tremor, unsteady gait, ataxia, confusion, drowsiness, and nystagmus. The combination is also known to produce additive antithyroid effects and carbamazepine-induced interstitial nephritis. However, addition of lithium mitigates carbamazepine-induced leukopenia and does not have any additive side effects on the hematopoietic system.

274. **Answer: A.** Blockade of the HERG potassium channel

HERG potassium channels are identified to initiate torsade de pointes.

275. **Answer: E.** None of the above

Lithium causes a relative depletion of myoinositol in the brain and subsequent regulation of PKC. Lithium inhibits G proteins via cAMP in the CNS, resulting in blocking of the neuronal activity that occurs in mania. Lithium is known to exchange readily with sodium and alters its transport both in nervous and muscular system.

276. **Answer: D.** CYP1A2

Smoking reduces clozapine level because smoking induces CYP1A2 and clozapine is a substrate for CYP1A2. Decreased clozapine level is the reason for this patient's relapse.

277. **Answer: E.** None of the above

Akathisia can be managed by lowering the neuroleptic dose, and initiation of ß-blockers or benzodiazepines is a preferred choice; however, antihistamines and anticholinergic agents have a role as well.

278. **Answer: B.** Increased risk for depression and suicide from her acne medication

Isotretinoin is recommended in the treatment of severe cystic acne. Literature reports that bipolar patients treated with isotretinoin for acne, even with ongoing medication management are at risk for worsening affective symptoms, including suicidal ideation. There is no DDI between isotretinoin and divalproex sodium.

279. **Answer: A.** Serotonin 5-HT$_2$A receptor

Trazodone has a great affinity for 5-HT$_2$A receptor and a moderate affinity for 5-HT$_1$A receptors.

280. **Answer: E.** All of the above

Depot paliperidone palmitate is efficacious for the acute and maintenance treatment of schizophrenia and is well tolerated. Unlike depot risperidone, it does not require refrigeration or reconstitution, can be administered monthly instead of biweekly, and does not require supplementation with oral antipsychotics. Olanzapine depot preparation requires a postinjection 3-hour observation that is not required with paliperidone palmitate.

281. **Answer: E.** Aripiprazole

Concurrent use of carbamazepine and divalproex sodium may result in carbamazepine toxicity and/or decreased divalproex sodium effectiveness. When coadministered with lamotrigine, it may result in lamotrigine toxicity and increases the risk of life-threatening rashes. Concurrent use of divalproex sodium and aspirin may result in increased free VPA concentrations. Similarly, coadministration of risperidone and divalproex sodium may result in increased plasma concentration of VPA. No DDI is reported between aripiprazole and divalproex sodium.

282. **Answer: B.** 20 mg/kg/day

Divalproex sodium is an effective antimanic agent and has evidence for preventing recurrence of bipolar disorder. Divalproex sodium 20 mg/kg/day when administered as a loading dose results in rapid resolution of manic symptoms.

283. **Answer: E.** None of the above

There is no contraindication or DDI between levothyroxine and propranolol. Concurrent use of clonidine and propranolol may result in acute hypertension and increased risk of sinus bradycardia. Propranolol when used with haloperidol may result in an increased risk of hypotension and cardiac arrest. Thioridazine when combined with propranolol may result in an increased risk of thioridazine toxicity and cardiotoxicity.

284. **Answer: E.** All of the above

MAOI is contraindicated in hepatic disease, renal insufficiency, CHF, and pheochromocytoma.

285. **Answer: B.** Formation of free radicals during microsomal metabolism of VPA

VPA is a category D drug in pregnancy. Even though the precise mechanism of VPA induced teratogenicity is not known, it is believed that the formation of free radicals during microsomal metabolism of valproate causes fetal anomalies.

286. **Answer: C.** Antagonism at muscarinic receptors

Asenapine, an antipsychotic medication approved for the treatment of schizophrenia, is an antagonist at the D_2 and 5-HT$_2$A receptors. It antagonizes adrenergic receptors but has no affinity for muscarinic receptors.

287. **Answer: C.** Clonazepam

Clonazepam is frequently used as an adjuvant to lithium in the treatment of mania.

288. **Answer: E.** None of the above

Heatstroke, serotonin syndrome, withdrawal from dopamine agonists, and malignant hyperthermia can mimic NMS.

289. **Answer: E.** All of the above

VPA exposure during pregnancy results in fetal/neonatal hepatotoxicity, coagulopathies, neural tube defects, and hypoglycemia.

290. **Answer: C.** >9 μg per ml

Most adverse effects of carbamazepine are correlated with the plasma concentration >9 μg per ml.

291. **Answer: A.** Whites

The highest percentage of CYP2D6 isoenzyme poor metabolizers is among Caucasians. Thus, poor metabolizers pose the risk of toxicity at therapeutic doses. Conversely, fast metabolizers are nonresponders at therapeutic doses.

292. **Answer: A.** Guide detoxification from barbiturates

Pentobarbital challenge test is used to guide detoxification from barbiturates. This involves administration of pentobarbital 200 mg orally and monitoring the clinical response of the patient. On the basis of the tolerance of the patient, 24-hour pentobarbital requirement is estimated and then converted to phenobarbital. Pentobarbital 100 mg equals 30 mg of phenobarbital.

293. **Answer: C.** Lithium has mild proserotonergic and adrenergic effects

Lithium is a mood stabilizer that is FDA approved for the treatment of manic episode and maintenance therapy of bipolar disorder. It is almost entirely excreted unchanged by the kidney (89% to 98%) and is not metabolized by the liver. Lithium has mild proserotonergic effects but no adrenergic effect. Lithium is a naturally occurring cation.

294. **Answer: E.** All of the above

Concurrent use of SJW, paroxetine, sertraline, or duloxetine with tamoxifen may result in reduced tamoxifen effectiveness.

295. **Answer: B.** Thioridazine

Thioridazine causes the most QTc prolongation at therapeutic doses. Haloperidol causes the least QTc prolongation at therapeutic doses.

296. **Answer: A.** Desvenlafaxine

Desvenlafaxine has minimal interaction with the CYP system. This may reduce potential DDIs. Duloxetine acts as both a substrate and an inhibitor of CYP2D6. Atomoxetine is primarily metabolized by the CYP2D6. Modafinil has been shown to inhibit CYP2C19 activity, and it is partially metabolized by the CYP3A4 isoenzyme.

297. **Answer: C.** Sympathomimetic effects

Pindolol is a nonselective β-blocker with partial β-adrenergic receptor agonist activity. Its sympathomimetic property acts as an augmentation agent in the treatment of depression.

298. **Answer: C.** Premature ejaculation

Dopamine blockade causes adverse effects such as galactorrhea, NMS, and bone loss.

299. **Answer: A.** Olanzapine

The CATIE trial concluded that the greatest body weight gain was observed with olanzapine.

300. **Answer: A.** Nonspecific T wave changes

Lithium at therapeutic doses can cause nonspecific T wave changes. No cases of torsades de pointes are reported with lithium use. Cardiotoxicity is uncommon with lithium overdose. ST segment elevation is reported in a case report, but it is rare.

301. **Answer: E.** All of the above

Carbamazepine, a folic acid antagonist, is an FDA category D drug. It is known to increase the risk of neural tube, cardiovascular, and urinary tract defects. Folate deficiency caused by carbamazepine is implicated in carbamazepine-induced teratogenesis. Hypoplasia of the nose, fingernails, ambiguous genitalia, congenital heart disease, cleft lip, congenital hip dislocation, and neural tube defects such as meningomyelocele, spina bifida, and inguinal hernia have been reported with carbamazepine use during pregnancy.

302. **Answer: D.** 2% to 3.5%

Ebstein anomaly is a congenital heart malformation, characterized by the downward displacement of the septal and posterior tricuspid valve leaflets, right ventricular dysfunction, and tricuspid regurgitation. In general population, the incidence of Ebstein anomaly is 0.005%, and its incidence is increased to 2.7% in the group of lithium-exposed babies.

303. **Answer: E.** Fluoxetine

Some antidepressants are known to lower seizure threshold and significantly increase the risk of seizures. Notable are bupropion, maprotiline, and clomipramine. However, with SSRIs or mirtazapine, the risk of seizure is not much different from the risk of seizure in the general population. In the clinical vignette, an SSRI such as fluoxetine would be a reasonable first choice for treating depression. Although phenelzine is not associated with a significantly elevated risk of seizures, MAOIs are usually not the first choice in depression because they require strict dietary restrictions.

304. **Answer: C.** Discontinue phenelzine, wait for 2 weeks, and then start tranylcypromine

Concurrent use of phenelzine and tranylcypromine may result in hypertensive crisis. Phenelzine, an irreversible nonselective monoamine inhibitor, takes up to 2 weeks to regenerate normal levels of MAO, after discontinuation.

305. **Answer: C.** Haloperidol

Haloperidol causes the least QTc prolongation at therapeutic doses.

306. **Answer: B.** Tranylcypromine

Tranylcypromine, a nonselective MAOI, is an activating agent and can be used in the management of anergic depressed patient.

307. **Answer: B.** Mirtazapine

Mirtazapine is the preferred drug in the management of this patient. All other antidepressants may be used, but mirtazapine's appetite-stimulating properties coupled with sedating effect make it an advantageous choice in this case.

308. **Answer: A.** It is partial agonist at $5\text{-HT}_1\text{A}$ receptor

Vilazodone is new antidepressant that FDA approved for the treatment of major depression; it is an SSRI and partial agonist at $5\text{-HT}_1\text{A}$ receptor. Vilazodone bioavailability increases with food, and the recommended dose of vilazodone 40 mg is once daily.

309. **Answer: C.** Doxepin

Doxepin is a TCA with significant antihistaminergic activity and is the drug that is used for the treatment of insomnia comorbid with depression and also used in dermatologic conditions characterized by pruritus and chronic itching.

310. **Answer: B.** Zaleplon

Zaleplon is a benzodiazepine receptor agonist with a very short half-life of 1 hour. Temazepam has a half-life between 10 and 15 hours, eszopiclone about 6 hours, and triazolam between 2 and 4.5 hours.

311. **Answer: D.** Paroxetine

Among the SSRIs, paroxetine has the highest likelihood of a discontinuation syndrome. Gradual taper of paroxetine is recommended over several days and in some cases even weeks. Elimination half-life of paroxetine is about 15 to 21 hours.

312. **Answer: D.** Carefully review pharmacy refill records for possible medication noncompliance

These symptoms are suggestive of antidepressant discontinuation syndrome. Symptoms such as mood lability, anxiety, dizziness, headache, fatigue, sleep disturbances, and GI tract complaints are common. This is especially common with venlafaxine. Pathologic crying and laughter and mood changes can be seen in stroke; however, the presenting symptoms do not support this possibility. Increasing the dose of olanzapine with divalproate is not the most appropriate management strategy at this time.

313. **Answer: B.** Hypothyroidism

Lithium suppresses thyroid functions that lead to subclinical or overt hypothyroidism in about 20% of patients. In this situation, it is not recommended to discontinue lithium, but hypothyroidism can be treated with thyroid replacement therapy. Hyperthyroidism, hypocalcemia, hypoparathyroidism, and hypoglycemia are rare side effects of lithium.

314. **Answer: C.** Paroxetine

Patient has symptoms of PMDD, characterized by mood swings, anger, irritability, and depressive symptoms around menstrual cycle. Paroxetine is used for the treatment of PMDD. Paroxetine can be used continuously or intermittently during the luteal phase of the menstrual cycle. Other agents listed are not used in the management of PMDD.

315. **Answer: C.** Lithium carbonate

Patient's symptoms are consistent with bipolar disorder. Bipolar disorder is managed with mood stabilizers. Antidepressant monotherapy can worsen bipolar disorder.

316. **Answer: D.** Prazosin

Prazosin is an α-adrenergic receptor antagonist, which also has vasodilator effect. The drug is being studied for nightmares and PTSD. Priapism can develop during treatment with prazosin. None of the other drugs listed have priapism as an adverse effect.

317. **Answer: C.** Nortriptyline

This is a classical presentation of TCA toxicity. TCA toxicity causes anticholinergic and antihistaminergic symptoms. TCA interferes with cardiac conduction system. Management of TCA toxicity includes hospitalization, cardiac monitoring, and sodium bicarbonate administration. If sodium bicarbonate fails, then lidocaine is indicated.

318. **Answer: A.** Alprazolam

Abrupt discontinuation of alprazolam produces withdrawal symptoms that include life-threatening seizures. Alprazolam has very short half-life when compared with other benzodiazepines. Other drugs listed have long half-life and have little risk of withdrawal symptoms.

319. **Answer: B.** Lithium carbonate

Treatment with lithium exacerbates psoriasis vulgaris within few months of the initiation of treatment. The exact mechanism for this exacerbation is not known. However, it may warrant discontinuation of lithium and to start an alternate mood stabilizer.

320. **Answer: B.** Clozapine

Clozapine has the least liability for extrapyramidal side effects among atypical neuroleptic agents.

321. **Answer: E.** None of the above

Higher doses are required to treat OCD. SSRIs have a flat dose–response curve unlike positive dose–response curve in venlafaxine. It is safe to use a different SSRI on a patient with a history of allergy to one SSRI because they are structurally distinct. PMDD responds well to SSRI treatment during late luteal phase.

322. **Answer: E.** All of the above

Risperidone microspheres start releasing significant amount of drug, 3 weeks after the injection. Hence, supplementation with oral antipsychotic must be continued for the first 3 weeks of therapy. When dose adjustment is made, clinical effects are expected after 3 weeks, following the injection at higher dose. Steady plasma concentrations are achieved after the fourth injection.

323. **Answer: E.** All of the above

Carbamazepine and VPA decreases olanzapine plasma concentrations. Fluvoxamine may increase olanzapine concentration and thus increasing the risk of olanzapine adverse effects. Olanzapine injections are only for IM use and should not be given intravenously. PDSS results from probable accidental intravascular injection of olanzapine long-acting preparation.

324. **Answer: A.** Inducing the CYP3A4 isoenzyme

SJW is a CYP3A4 inducer. Thus, it increases the metabolism of estrogen resulting in decreased efficacy of contraceptives. SJW may increase the metabolism of estrogen through intestinal p-glycoprotein metabolism.

325. **Answer: C.** Pimozide

Trifluoperazine (Stelazine), thiothixene (Navane), haloperidol, and pimozide are high-potency antipsychotics.

326. **Answer: E.** All of the above

Calorie and psychotherapy are proven to be efficacious for anorexia nervosa, and no pharmacotherapy is proven to be efficacious for anorexia nervosa. SSRIs are the first-line treatment for bulimia nervosa. Fluoxetine has shown to be effective in reducing binge eating and purging in bulimic women. The recommended dose of fluoxetine for bulimia nervosa is 60 mg per day on day 1. It was tolerated well, and perhaps fluoxetine is the only medication approved by FDA for bulimia. First-line treatment for binge eating disorder is uncertain.

327. **Answer: D.** Tetrabenazine

Ms. C has Huntington disease, an autosomal dominant neurodegenerative disorder. In normal individuals, CAG repeats are between 10 and 35, but in patients with Huntington disease, it is repeated up to 36 and 120 times. Tetrabenazine is approved by FDA for treatment of Huntington chorea. Neuroleptics and benzodiazepines have a role in the treatment of reducing chorea.

328. **Answer: C.** Benztropine

Neuroleptic-induced dystonia is managed with anticholinergics such as benztropine. Antihistamines can be used as well. β-Blockers such as propranolol is indicated in neuroleptic-induced acute akathisia.

329. **Answer: E.** All of the above

Carbamazepine, SJW, modafinil, and topiramate may result in reduced contraceptive efficacy. Patients should be managed with an alternative nonhormonal contraception method.

330. **Answer: C.** Fluoxetine

SSRIs are known to delay ejaculation as one of the adverse sexual side effects. This is mediated by increasing the central serotonin (5-HT) neurotransmission and postsynaptic activation of 5-HT. This adverse effect may be used to treat premature ejaculation.

331. **Answer: D.** Moclobemide

Moclobemide is a selective and reversible MAO-A inhibitor. Phenelzine, tranylcypromine, and isocarboxazid are nonselective MAOI. Selegiline is an MAO-B inhibitor.

332. **Answer: D.** Lamotrigine

By measuring the plasma drug level of lithium, VPA, nortriptyline, and clozapine, optimal efficacious dosing may be assessed. Serum level of lamotrigine is not measured.

333. **Answer: E.** All of the above

Risperidone increases the prolactin level the most among the atypical neuroleptics. Aripiprazole can be used to normalize neuroleptic-induced prolactin elevation. Clozapine has the least effect on prolactin therapy, and typical antipsychotics are associated with persistently elevated prolactin level.

334. **Answer: D.** Lifelong antidepressant maintenance treatment is indicated for this patient

APA major depressive disorder guidelines recommend that maintenance treatment be considered for those with risk factors for MDD and/or with a history of three or more prior depressive episodes or chronic or severe illness. Monthly ECTs are indicated for patients with treatment-resistant depression and who have responded to an acute course of 8 to 15 ECT sessions.

335. **Answer: D.** Buspirone

Buspirone is an approved medication in the treatment of GAD. It is not sedating and has no abuse liability.

336. **Answer: B.** Physostigmine

Physostigmine is an indirect-acting parasympathomimetic drug and used in the management of anticholinergic toxicity. Phentolamine is an α-adrenergic blocker and used in the management of hypertensive crisis. Flumazenil is used in benzodiazepine overdose.

337. **Answer: E.** VPA

When combined with VPA, it may increase the elimination half-life of lamotrigine leading to lamotrigine toxicity as well as increase in the risk of life-threatening rash. Oral contraceptives may decrease the level of lamotrigine. No DDI is reported between lamotrigine and bupropion, alprazolam, or fluoxetine.

338. **Answer: C.** Hypotension

Concurrent use of vardenafil and prazosin may result in potentiation of hypotensive effects.

339. **Answer: B.** Patients on lithium should reduce their sodium intake

Patients on lithium are educated to continue their usual sodium intake because low intake raises the lithium level and high intake drops the level.

340. **Answer: D.** Antipsychotic–smoking CYP-mediated interaction

Smoking affects the metabolism of various psychiatric medications by inducing enzymes in the CYP1A2 subtype. Smoking can lower serum levels of antipsychotics such as olanzapine and clozapine by almost 50%. Hence, in patients who resume smoking after a period of abstinence experience reduced plasma levels leading to breakthrough symptoms. Conversely, after successful smoking cessation, the subsequent lack of enzyme induction can lead to drug toxicity with olanzapine and clozapine. Although there have been reports of bupropion-induced psychosis, this is quite rare.

341. **Answer: B.** Ziprasidone

The CATIE trial concluded that body weight decrease was observed with ziprasidone.

342. **Answer: E.** All of the above

Triazolam may result in increased triazolam concentrations and potential triazolam toxicity when combined with nefazodone, ketoconazole, amprenavir, or efavirenz.

343. **Answer: D.** Hypertensive crisis associated with MAOI and tyramine ingestion

Phentolamine is an α-adrenergic blocker and is used in the management of hypertensive crisis.

344. **Answer: E.** All of the above

Thioridazine is known to cause retinal pigmentation and visual impairment that usually develops within 2 to 8 weeks after initiation of the treatment. Even after thioridazine is discontinued, pigmentary changes may progress but visual impairment usually improves. Leukopenia and agranulocytosis are the most common hematologic side effects associated with thioridazine use. Retrograde ejaculation and torsades de pointes are reported side effects of thioridazine.

345. **Answer: B.** Metoclopramide

Torticollis, an acute dystonic reaction, is secondary to metoclopramide. The most common type of extrapyramidal reactions associated with metoclopramide is acute dystonic reaction, which is estimated to be around 0.2%. It usually occurs during the first 24 to 48 hours of treatment. It is managed with either diphenhydramine or benztropine.

346. **Answer: C.** Sertraline

SSRIs are safe in post-MI patients. Among the SSRIs, sertraline has the most data, and fluoxetine should be avoided because of potential for DDIs. TCAs are known to be cardiotoxic. Venlafaxine can be problematic in cases of uncontrolled hypertension. MAOIs should be avoided in the post-MI period.

347. **Answer: C.** Combination of an antidepressant and an antipsychotic

Depression with psychotic features is managed with a combination of an antidepressant and an antipsychotic medication.

348. **Answer: C.** Quetiapine

Quetiapine has evidence in treating psychotic symptoms in a patient with Parkinson disease. Its favorable profile on extrapyramidal side effects makes it a better choice among Parkinson disease (PD) patients. Similarly, clozapine is preferred as well.

349. **Answer: C.** Muscle rigidity, hyperthermia, and altered mental status

Initiation of linezolid in this patient may result in serotonin syndrome. Serotonin neurons play a role in thermoregulation; an increase in serotonergic activity can lead to thermoregulatory dysfunction that explains the fever and shivering seen in serotonin syndrome. Besides supportive measures, prompt initiation of cyproheptadine is recommended in the treatment of serotonin syndrome.

350. **Answer: C.** Flumazenil

When mixed overdose with TCAs is suspected, flumazenil is contraindicated. Flumazenil is thought to unmask TCA-induced seizure because flumazenil antagonizes anticonvulsive effects of coingested benzodiazepine. Thus, flumazenil can cause convulsions.

351. **Answer: E.** None of the above

Oxcarbazepine, an anticonvulsant, is the 10-keto derivative of carbamazepine. The mechanism of action of oxcarbazepine is similar to that of carbamazepine. Hyponatremia is a concern with oxcarbazepine therapy and not hypernatremia. The adverse effects profile of both drugs is similar with respect to enzyme induction and hematologic effects.

352. **Answer: A.** Increase risk of myopathy

Concurrent use of risperidone and simvastatin may increase the bio-availability of simvastatin and increase the risk of myopathy and rhabdomyolysis. This is secondary to a DDI mediated by CYP3A4.

353. **Answer: A.** Nefazodone

Nefazodone is devoid of any sexual side effects.

354. **Answer: A.** Abstinence from alcohol during the course of Depakote therapy

VPA has a black box warning for hepatotoxicity. Fatal cases have been reported, and patients need to be warned about this adverse effect. Onset of hepatotoxicity is reported during the first 6 months of the treatment.

355. **Answer: C.** Aripiprazole

Antipsychotic blockade of D_2 receptors in the anterior pituitary gland releases the inhibitory action of dopamine and increases prolactin secretion. Elevated prolactin levels during antipsychotic therapy can lead to menstrual irregularities, sexual dysfunction, galactorrhea, and low bone mineral density. Aripiprazole is unique among the antipsychotics because it has partial agonistic effects on the D_2 receptors and thus not associated with elevated prolactin levels. In fact, adjunctive aripiprazole is clinically useful to normalize elevated prolactin levels during antipsychotic therapy.

356. **Answer: B.** Antipsychotic-induced weight gain is solely correlated to the affinity of the antipsychotic drug for histamine receptors

The precise molecular mechanisms responsible for antipsychotic drug-induced weight gain are unknown. Currently postulated mechanisms include antagonism of $5\text{-}HT_2C$ receptors and histamine H_1 receptor, and interactions involving appetite and energy homeostatic peptides such as leptin, ghrelin, and adiponectin.

357. **Answer: A.** Lithium

VPA has black box warning for hepatic failure. Hepatitis, cholestatic jaundice, and abnormal liver function tests are reported with olanzapine and carbamazepine.

358. **Answer: A.** The mechanism of VPA-induced thrombocytopenia is believed to be an immune destruction of platelets by VPA

Low platelet counts and thrombocytopenia have been associated with VPA treatment. These side effects are seen at higher doses of VPA (VPA serum level above 80 μg per ml), more common among women and the elderly and those with low baseline platelet counts. VPA-induced low platelet counts or thrombocytopenia usually runs a benign course and can be managed by close monitoring of platelet counts and dose reduction alone. Because VPA-induced thrombocytopenia develops gradually over a course of time, this suggests a bone marrow suppression effect mediated by VPA, rather than an immune-mediated destruction of platelets (associated with rapid development of thrombocytopenia).

359. **Answer: E.** Bipolar disorder, manic episode

Topiramate is FDA approved for the management of seizure disorder and migraine prophylaxis. It has evidence for the management of eating disorder and alcohol dependence but not for bipolar disorder, manic episode.

360. **Answer: A.** GI

GI adverse effects are the most common side effects of SSRI therapy.

361. **Answer: B.** Sertraline

Sertraline is known to have dopaminergic activity. Neurochemical differences among the SSRIs account for the differences in clinical response in the treatment of depression.

362. **Answer: A.** Bipolar disorder, depressed phase

Aripiprazole is approved for the treatment of bipolar disorder, manic or mixed phase but not for the depressed phase.

363. **Answer: D.** Quetiapine

Quetiapine is approved as a monotherapy for bipolar disorder, depressed phase.

364. **Answer: C.** PTSD

Therapeutic lag with SSRIs in the management of PTSD can be as long as 8 to 12 weeks as opposed to 4 to 6 weeks in the management of MDD.

365. **Answer: D.** Clozapine

Salivation is seen in 31% of patients receiving clozapine therapy. Clozapine-induced sialorrhea may be profuse, and dosage reduction may help. Mechanism of action proposed includes muscarinic M_4-receptor stimulation by clozapine, antagonism at α_2-adrenergic receptor, and interference with the normal swallowing reflex.

366. **Answer: E.** Paroxetine

Paroxetine is known for its anticholinergic property among the SSRIs.

367. **Answer: A.** SSRIs

An amotivational or apathy syndrome has been reported in several patients receiving SSRIs. Patients experiencing this side effect exhibit behavioral changes such as becoming indifferent toward work performance, exhibit impulsive and disinhibited behavior, or develop poor concentration and forgetful behavior. This side effect is often overlooked and missed. This side effect usually responds to dose reduction and/or switching antidepressant classes. Stimulants are typically used to manage symptoms of apathy.

Chapter 2

Pediatric Psychopharmacology

Questions

1. The atypical antipsychotic risperidone is U.S. Food and Drug Administration (FDA) approved for use in the management of children and adolescents with autistic disorder. Despite its overall efficacy, the drug has demonstrated minimal to no success in treating which of the following core symptoms of autism?

   A. Aggressive behavior

   B. Repetitive and stereotyped patterns of behavior

   C. Deficits in social interaction and communication

   D. Self-injurious behavior

   E. Hallucinations

2. What is the half-life of methylphenidate?

   A. 8 to 10 hours

   B. 6 to 8 hours

   C. 3 to 4 hours

   D. 1 to 2 hours

   E. 30 to 60 minutes

3. All of the following medications have role in Rx of tics EXCEPT:

    A. Haloperidol

    B. Pimozide

    C. Atomoxetine

    D. Clonidine

    E. Tetrabenazine

4. A 16-year-old boy is being seen in an outpatient clinic for schizophrenia following a recent inpatient first episode psychotic break. He was started on oral paliperidone during his hospitalization and is taking 3 mg once daily. His parents are very concerned that their son appears withdrawn and shows lack of interest. There are no active symptoms of psychosis. Which of the following interventions has highest priority at this time?

    A. Monitor for metabolic side effects of paliperidone by obtaining fasting lipid profile

    B. Conduct an Abnormal Involuntary Movement Scale test (AIMS) exam

    C. Assess for symptoms of major depression and consider antidepressant treatment

    D. Family and individual counseling about schizophrenia

    E. Assessment of social and educationally needs of the patient

5. Which of the following is used as a first-line agent in the treatment of enuresis?

    A. Venlafaxine

    B. Fluoxetine

    C. Imipramine

    D. Desmopressin

    E. Modafinil

6. All of following statements are true except regarding the use of clonidine in children EXCEPT:

    A. Clonidine is useful in the pharmacologic treatment of Tourette syndrome in children

    B. Sedation is most frequent and troublesome side effect of clonidine

    C. Personal history of cardiovascular disease is contraindication for starting clonidine therapy in children

    D. Clonidine should be titrated gradually, and dose can be increased every 2 to 3 days

    E. Clonidine has a long half-life, and it is administered orally once or twice a day

7. You are treating a 14-year-old adolescent female for symptoms of depression. The patient reports two trials with a selective serotonin reuptake inhibitor (SSRI) at maximum doses, that is, citalopram and fluoxetine along with weekly cognitive behavioral therapy. She continues to experience symptoms such as dysphoria, anhedonia, guilt, and poor concentration. She has no suicidal thought. Her school grades have been improved. There are no concerns regarding medication compliance. There is family history of depression on the paternal side and bipolar disorder on the maternal side. Which of the following will be most appropriate next step in the management of this patient?

    A. Reassess diagnosis; especially rule out bipolar disorder or co-morbid attention-deficit hyperactivity disorder (ADHD)

    B. Consider augmentation with lithium

    C. Consider augmentation with venlafaxine

    D. Consider augmentation with atypical antipsychotics

    E. All of the above

8. You are treating a 15-year-old adolescent boy for ADHD and comorbid depression. Based on careful history and assessment and other information, you determined that the depressive symptoms are a bigger problem compared with his ADHD. Which of the following management will be the most appropriate next step?

    A. Start bupropion for depression and ADHD

    B. Attempt a trial of fluoxetine

    C. Prescribe combination of fluoxetine and a stimulant such as methylphenidate

    D. Prescribe atomoxetine

    E. Start with methylphenidate monotherapy

9. A 10-year-old child is diagnosed with ADHD and prescribed methylphenidate. His symptoms improve as well as school grades improve significantly. His mother voices concerns regarding growth slowdown. All of the following statements regarding psychostimulant growth slowdown are true EXCEPT:

    A. Stimulant-induced appetite suppression and reduced caloric intake may play a role in growth retardation

    B. Stimulants may suppress growth hormone release

    C. Height and weight gain should be recorded once a year in patients receiving stimulants

    D. In the presence of height or weight velocity, dose reduction has no role and change to another class of medication must be carried out

    E. None of the above

10. Which of the following statements is true regarding the differences in drug metabolism between children and adults?

    A. Children have proportionally smaller liver tissue

    B. Children have slower hepatic drug metabolism

    C. Children have lower glomerular filtration rates

    D. Children may more rapidly excrete the drug that uses either hepatic or renal pathways

    E. All of the above

11. Which of the following statement is true regarding the pharmacologic treatment of ADHD symptoms among children and adolescents with intellectual disability?

    A. Risperidone should be the first line of treatment

    B. Stimulants should be the first line of treatment

    C. Combination of antipsychotic and stimulant is the standard of care

    D. Antidepressants should be the first line of treatment

    E. Anticonvulsants should be the first line of treatment

12. Which of the following statement is true regarding the pharmacotherapy of ADHD?

    A. Methylphenidate is approved for children ≥ 3 years

    B. Methylphenidate is approved for children ≥ 4 years

    C. Methylphenidate is approved for children ≥ 5 years

    D. Methylphenidate is approved for children ≥ 6 years

    E. Methylphenidate is approved for children ≥ 7 years

13. Which of the following statement is true regarding the pharmacotherapy of ADHD with amphetamine?

    A. Amphetamine is approved for children ≥3 years

    B. Amphetamine is approved for children ≥6 years

    C. Amphetamine can be safely used in a patient with hyperthyroidism

    D. Amphetamine can be safely used within a week following discontinuation of monoamine oxidase inhibitors (MAOIs)

    E. Amphetamine can be safely used in children with structural cardiac abnormalities

14. Among children, which of the following medications affects cardiovascular functioning and may prolong QTc even at therapeutic doses?

    A. Clonidine

    B. Thioridazine

    C. Tricyclic antidepressants

    D. Lithium

    E. All of the above

15. An 8-year-old male child was started on 20 μg intranasal desmopressin (1-desamino-8-D-arginine vasopressin [DDAVP]) for primary nocturnal enuresis. Which of the following is the most common side effect with intranasal desmopressin?

    A. Water intoxication

    B. Headache

    C. Epistaxis

    D. Abdominal pain

    E. Seizure

16. Which of the following medications is FDA approved for major depressive disorder (MDD) in adolescents?

    A. Citalopram

    B. Sertraline

    C. Escitalopram

    D. Paraxetine

    E. Fluvoxamine

17. Which of the following statements is true regarding the pharmacokinetics in children?

    A. Children have proportionally less total-body water than adults

    B. Children have higher plasma concentrations of hydrophilic drugs than adults

    C. Children have proportionally less adipose tissue than adults

    D. Children have lower plasma concentrations of lipophilic drugs than adults

    E. All of the above

18. β-Adrenergic agents are used in the management of aggression associated with which of the following conditions?

    A. Intermittent explosive disorder

    B. Traumatic brain injury

    C. Autism

    D. ADHD

    E. All of the above

19. Which of the following statements is not true regarding psychopharmacotherapy between children and adults?

    A. Psychopharmacotherapy in children is distinct from adults

    B. Metabolism of drugs differs between children and adults

    C. Efficacy and tolerability of psychotropic drugs differs between children and adults

    D. Abundant research data on pediatric psychopharmacology is available

    E. Treatment in child psychiatry is mostly multidisciplinary in nature

20. All of the following statements regarding dexmethylphenidate (Focalin) are true EXCEPT:

    A. Dexmethylphenidate is the active D-enantiomer of racemic methylphenidate

    B. For patients currently on methylphenidate, the recommended starting dose of dexmethylphenidate is half the total daily dose of racemic methylphenidate

    C. Dexmethylphenidate can be administered by sprinkling the capsule contents on a small amount of applesauce

    D. The difference in duration of action between dexmethylphenidate and methylphenidate is not clinically significant

    E. Studies indicate a more favorable adverse effect profile for dexmethylphenidate compared with methylphenidate

21. All of the following statements regarding lisdexamfetamine area true EXCEPT:

  A. It is a prodrug of dextroamphetamine

  B. Lisdexamfetamine is not metabolized by cytochrome P450 enzymes

  C. Lisdexamfetamine dimesylate has lower abuse potential

  D. The drug's short duration of action is a key determinant of its efficacy in school-going children with ADHD

  E. It is schedule II drug which means that automated refills are not allowed

22. Which of the following must be closely monitored during guanfacine therapy?

  A. Liver function test

  B. Renal function test

  C. Blood pressure

  D. Lipid panel

  E. Platelet count

23. Which of the following can be a potential risk factor for increased blood pressure and seizure in children taking atomoxetine?

  A. Coadministration of aripiprazole

  B. Coadministration of risperidone

  C. Coadministration of bupropion

  D. Slow CPY2D6 metabolizer

  E. All of the above

24. Which of the following medications has the strongest evidence for the management of aggression and self-injurious behavior in children with autism spectrum disorders?

    A. Methylphenidate

    B. Naltrexone

    C. Clonidine

    D. Lithium

    E. Fluoxetine

25. Which of the following statements is true regarding cardiovascular assessment and monitoring during pediatric ADHD pharmacotherapy?

    A. The American Heart Association requires a mandatory electrocardiogram (EKG) before starting stimulants in ADHD

    B. Clinical studies have demonstrated statistically significant changes in QTc parameters during pediatric ADHD pharmacotherapy with stimulants as well as nonstimulants

    C. The link between stimulants and sudden death in children is well established

    D. There is an FDA black box warning regarding cardiovascular fatalities associated with the use of stimulants in ADHD

    E. None of the above

26. Which of the following is true regarding α_2-adrenergic agonist therapy among children?

    A. Clonidine is used in the management of ADHD

    B. Clonidine is used in the management of tics

    C. Guanfacine is used in the management of Gilles de la Tourette syndrome

    D. Guanfacine is FDA-approved treatment for ADHD

    E. All of the above

27. A 16-year-old Caucasian girl was diagnosed with bipolar affective disorder, and she was started on a mood stabilizer about 6 months ago. During the follow-up visit, she complained about menstrual irregularities and weight gain. On examination, she has hirsutism and acne. She is not on any other medications. You suspect polycystic ovarian syndrome (PCOS). Which of the following mood stabilizers have been associated with the development of PCOS?

   A. Lithium

   B. Valproic acid

   C. Aripiprazole

   D. Ziprasidone

   E. None of the above

28. Which of the following is proven to be efficacious in the treatment of Tourette disorder?

   A. Methylphenidate

   B. Pimozide

   C. Clonazepam

   D. Propranolol

   E. Atomoxetine

29. A 10-year-old girl is diagnosed with ADHD. She has no significant medical history. Her family history is significant for long QT syndrome in her mother. You consider starting her on stimulant. What is the next best step in the management of this patient?

   A. Order an electrocardiogram

   B. Order an echocardiogram

   C. Request a 24-hour Holter monitoring

   D. Consult a pediatric cardiologist

   E. Start bupropion instead of a stimulant

30. All of the following are true regarding methylphenidate EXCEPT:

   A. The drug inhibits reuptake of dopamine and norepinephrine into presynaptic neurons

   B. It is inconclusive whether or not prolonged use of methylphenidate can significantly limit height and body weight

   C. Dexmethylphenidate (Focalin) is the D-enantiomer of methylphenidate

   D. The efficacy and safety of methylphenidate has not been established in patients <6 years of age

   E. Routine baseline EKGs are recommended before starting methylphenidate therapy

31. All of the following statements regarding methylphenidate transdermal system are true EXCEPT:

   A. The patch should be applied to the hip area and should be removed 6 hours after application

   B. The effect on average dissipates 3 hours after patch removal

   C. The transdermal formulation produces higher exposures of dexmethylphenidate compared with oral administration

   D. It is dosed once a day

   E. None of the above

32. Which of the following is the first-line pharmacotherapy for childhood anxiety disorder?

   A. Sertraline

   B. Lorazepam

   C. Imipramine

   D. Modafinil

   E. Venlafaxine

33. All of the following statements regarding atomoxetine are true EXCEPT:

A. FDA approved for ADHD

B. Middle insomnia is characteristic of noradrenergic rebound and might be expected during atomoxetine therapy

C. Atomoxetine has no effect on blood pressure and pulse when compared with stimulants

D. Atomoxetine has no abuse liability

E. Atomoxetine has black box warning for suicidal ideation in children and adolescents

34. Which of the following statement is true regarding neuroleptic-induced extrapyramidal side effects among children and adolescents?

A. Risk of extrapyramidal symptoms (EPS) increases with higher dose of aripiprazole

B. Quetiapine is associated with lower EPS

C. Sensitive than adults to EPS associated with atypical antipsychotics

D. Sensitive than adults to EPS associated with typical antipsychotics

E. All of the above

35. Which of the following is true regarding management of insomnia in pediatrics patients?

A. Zaleplon because of its shorter half-life is the preferred agent

B. There is no FDA-approved agent for the management of insomnia

C. Nonpharmacologic therapy combined with pharmacotherapy yields the optimal response

D. Cognitive behavioral therapy has very limited role in the management of insomnia

E. All of the above

36. All of the following SSRIs are FDA-approved treatment for obsessive-compulsive disorder (OCD) EXCEPT:

 A. Fluoxetine

 B. Fluvoxamine

 C. Sertraline

 D. Citalopram

 E. None of the above

37. Which of the following treatment is associated with better outcome in primary nocturnal enuresis?

 A. Imipramine

 B. Desmopressin

 C. Modafanil

 D. Bell and pad conditioning

 E. All of the above

Answers

1. **Answer: C.** Deficits in social interaction and communication

Risperidone is FDA approved in children older than 5 years with autism and irritability. It has demonstrated efficacy in treating aggression, irritability, repetitive, stereotyped patterns of behavior and self-injurious behavior in children with autism spectrum disorders. However, it has modest benefits in improving deficits in social interaction and communication. In such cases, behavioral intervention is the best option.

2. **Answer: C.** 3 to 4 hours

Half-life of methylphenidate is about 3 to 4 hours.

3. **Answer: C.** Atomoxetine

Atomoxetine, a selective norepinephrine inhibitor, is a nonstimulant alternative treatment because ADHD does not have a role in the management of tics. It was marketed that it is safe to use in children with comorbid tics or Tourette syndrome; however, atomoxetine is reported to exacerbate and precipitate tics in children with ADHD.

4. **Answer: C.** Assess for symptoms of major depression and consider antidepressant treatment

Adolescent schizophrenia is a devastating illness with greater clinical severity and poor outcome. Adolescent schizophrenia is frequently accompanied by negative symptoms as well as depressive symptoms. There is also a high risk of suicide and a major cause of death in schizophrenia. This is especially true in the immediate aftermath of inpatient hospitalization.

5. **Answer: D.** Desmopressin

Desmopressin is the first-line treatment for primary nocturnal enuresis. Imipramine because of its toxicity during overdose and cardiac monitoring is used for refractory cases.

6. **Answer: E.** Clonidine has a long half-life, and it is administered orally once or twice a day

Clonidine has a very short half-life, hence administered three to four times daily. Multiple doses can be avoided by using transdermal formulation of clonidine. In addition to slow titration, it is recommended to gradually taper off the drug during discontinuation.

7. **Answer: A.** Reassess diagnosis; especially rule out bipolar disorder or comorbid ADHD

When managing depression in the pediatric setting, it is important to reassess and confirm diagnosis. It is important to rule out comorbid conditions like bipolar disorder, ADHD, posttraumatic stress disorder first before augmentation. Although venlafaxine, bupropion, lithium, and atypical antipsychotic have not been studied in this population, these medications can be used for augmentation.

8. **Answer: B.** Attempt a trial of fluoxetine

In the treatment of comorbid ADHD and major depression, it is important to identify the bigger problem and target therapy toward it. In this case, a trial of fluoxetine might be efficacious for both set of symptoms.

9. **Answer: C.** Height and weight gain should be recorded once a year in patients receiving stimulants

Methylphenidate suppresses linear growth in child and adolescents. So their height and weight should be closely monitored for growth suppression periodically. Physicians interrupt methylphenidate treatment on holidays, summer, and even weekends for growth catch-up.

10. **Answer: D.** Children may more rapidly excrete the drug that uses either hepatic or renal pathways

Children have proportionally more liver tissue than adults. This results in more rapid hepatic drug metabolism than adults and rapid elimination of drugs that use hepatic pathways. Similarly children have higher glomerular filtration rates than adults which may result in rapid excretion of drugs that use renal pathways.

11. **Answer: B.** Stimulants should be the first line of treatment

Use of stimulants such as, methylphenidate, dextroamphetamine, and mixed amphetamine salts are the first-line treatments for ADHD symptoms in children and adolescents with intellectual disability. Current recommendation is a trial of stimulants before a trial of an antipsychotic agent. Risperidone is FDA approved for the treatment of irritability in children with autism.

12. **Answer: D.** Methylphenidate is approved for children ≥6 years

Methylphenidate is not recommended for children younger than 6 years because safety and efficacy have not been established.

13. **Answer: A.** Amphetamine is approved for children ≥3 years

Amphetamine is not recommended for children younger than 3 years because safety and efficacy have not been established. It is contraindicated in hyperthyroidism. Amphetamine should not be used during or within 2 weeks following discontinuation of MAOIs because the combination can cause hypertensive crisis.

14. **Answer: E.** All of the above

First-generation and second-generation antipsychotics, tricyclic antidepressants, and lithium affect cardiovascular functioning. Clonidine and guanfacine are known to have cardiovascular side effects. Cardiovascular monitoring is recommended while children are treated with these agents.

15. **Answer: B.** Headache

Headache is the most common side effect with intranasal desmopressin. Epistaxis is reported with intranasal desmopressin. Water intoxication presents with abdominal pain and hyponatremia. Untreated hyponatremia may result in seizures; however, these side effects are not very common.

16. **Answer: C.** Escitalopram

Escitalopram and fluoxetine are the two antidepressants currently approved by FDA for the treatment of pediatric depression.

17. **Answer: C.** Children have proportionally less adipose tissue than adults

Total-body water in children is proportionally higher than that in adults. This may lead to lower plasma concentrations of hydrophilic drugs. However, children may have higher concentrations of some lipophilic drugs because they have proportionally less adipose tissue than adults.

18. **Answer: E.** All of the above

β-Adrenergic agents are used in the management of aggression associated with intermittent explosive disorder, traumatic brain injury, autistic disorder, ADHD, and Tourette syndrome.

19. Answer: D. Abundant research data on pediatric psychopharmacology is available

There is little data available on pediatric psychopharmacology. Psycho-pharmacotherapy in children is distinct from adults and their metabolism of drugs is different from adults. Efficacy and tolerability of psychotropic drugs differs between children and adults. Treatment in child psychiatry is mostly multidisciplinary in nature.

20. Answer: E. Studies indicate a more favorable adverse effect profile for dexmethylphenidate compared to methylphenidate

Dexmethylphenidate (Focalin) is the D-enantiomer of methylpheni-date. It is a norepinephrine-dopamine reuptake inhibitor commonly used in the treatment for ADHD. The capsules can be administered by sprinkling their contents on the applesauce or pudding. For patients currently on methylphenidate, the recommended starting dose of dex-methylphenidate is half the total daily dose of racemic methylphenidate. The difference in duration of action between dexmethylphenidate and methylphenidate is not clinically significant, and both agents are admin-istered twice daily at similar intervals. Studies have not indicated a more favorable adverse effect profile for dexmethylphenidate compared to methylphenidate

21. Answer: D. The drug's short duration of action is a key determinant of its efficacy in school-going children with ADHD

Lisdexamfetamine is a prodrug, which is rapidly absorbed and converted to the active drug dextroamphetamine. It is not metabolized by cyto-chrome P450 isoenzymes. It is schedule II drug which means that auto-mated refills are not allowed. Lisdexamfetamine dimesylate has lower abuse potential resulting from multiple factors such as being a prodrug, longer T_{max},m and slow-release preparation. Lisdexamfetamine provides a long-acting duration of effect that is consistent throughout the day, which is the key determinant of its efficacy in school-going children with ADHD.

22. Answer: C. Blood pressure

Guanfacine therapy is associated with a drop in blood pressure and de-creased heart rate. Therefore periodic monitoring of blood pressure and heart rate is indicated.

23. **Answer: D.** Slow CPY2D6 metabolizer

When atomoxetine is administered in poor metabolizers, plasma concentration of atomoxetine is raised to 5-fold, thus increasing the risk of raising the blood pressure as well as seizure risk.

24. **Answer: A.** Methylphenidate

Aggression and self-injury are seen in autism, and these symptoms are treated with a broad range of pharmacologic approaches. Among the agents listed, there is strong evidence for methylphenidate in managing these symptoms. Risperidone is FDA approved in children older than 5 years with autism and irritability.

25. **Answer: E.** None of the above

There has been no definitive causality established between serious cardiovascular events and sudden death in children, adolescents, and adults treated with stimulants. Except for cases where there is a patient and family history of sudden or unexplained death and/or sudden cardiac death, there are no indications for an either an EKG or cardiology consultation before starting stimulant therapy.

26. **Answer: E.** All of the above

Clonidine is used in the management of ADHD and tics. Guanfacine is FDA approved for ADHD. It has a role in the management of Gilles de la Tourette's syndrome.

27. **Answer: B.** Valproic acid

There is a growing body of literature that supports the association of valproic acid and PCOS. Current recommendation is to avoid valproic acid in teenagers and young women of childbearing age.

28. **Answer: B.** Pimozide

Pimozide is FDA-approved treatment of Gilles de la Tourette syndrome. Methylphenidate and atomoxetine are reported to exacerbate and precipitate tics.

29. **Answer: A.** Order an electrocardiogram

Medications used in the management of ADHD have not been proven to cause heart conditions or sudden cardiac death. Current recommendations for children and adolescents being prescribed stimulants include a careful review of personal and family cardiovascular history and physical examination. In the presence of risk factors for cardiac disease, further assessment, including ECG and a referral to a pediatric cardiologist, should be considered.

30. **Answer: E.** Routine baseline EKGs are recommended before starting methylphenidate therapy

Methylphenidate blocks the reuptake of norepinephrine and dopamine into the presynaptic neuron, thus increasing the concentrations of these monoamines in the extraneural space. FDA-approved indications do not support the use of this drug in children younger than 6 years. EKGs are only indicated in cases of personal or family history of cardiac conditions.

31. **Answer: A.** The patch should be applied to the hip area and should be removed 6 hours after application

Methylphenidate is a racemic mixture which is composed of D- and L-enantiomers. The D-enantiomer is more pharmacologically active. The transdermal formulation produces higher exposures of dexmethylphenidate compared with oral administration because the transdermal administration of methylphenidate undergoes much less first-pass effect than the oral preparation. Methylphenidate transdermal system, which is dosed once a day, should be applied topically 2 hours before needed effect, and it should be removed 9 hours after application. The effect on average dissipates 3 hours after patch removal.

32. **Answer: A.** Sertraline

SSRIs are the first-line treatment for childhood anxiety disorder.

33. **Answer: C.** Atomoxetine has no effect on blood pressure and pulse when compared with stimulants

Atomoxetine is FDA approved for the management of ADHD. Atomoxetine has black box warning for suicidal ideation in children and adolescents. It does not have abuse liability. Middle insomnia is characteristic of noradrenergic rebound and might be expected during atomoxetine therapy as opposed to initial insomnia with stimulants. Atomoxetine is reported to increase systolic and diastolic blood pressure and may cause palpitations.

34. **Answer: E.** All of the above

Risk of EPS increases with higher dose of aripiprazole. Just like adults, quetiapine is associated with lower EPS. Children and adolescents are sensitive than adults to EPS associated with both atypical and typical antipsychotics.

35. **Answer: B.** There is no FDA-approved agent for the management of insomnia

Nonpharmacologic therapy such as behavioral interventions and cognitive therapy are the first-line management of childhood and adolescent insomnia. There is no FDA-approved treatment for the management of insomnia.

36. **Answer: D.** Citalopram

Fluoxetine, sertraline, and fluvoxamine are FDA-approved treatments for the management of OCD.

37. **Answer: D.** Bell and pad conditioning

Literature indicates that at 12 months follow-up, even after termination of the treatment, bell and pad conditioning is better in preventing relapse of enuresis when compared with imipramine and desmopressin.

Chapter 3

Geriatric Psychopharmacology

Questions

1. You are treating a 72-year-old man for major depressive disorder (MDD). You start him on citalopram 10 mg to which he responds fairly well. Which of the following electrolyte abnormalities is a rare but dangerous side effect associated with citalopram therapy?

    A. Hypocalcemia

    B. Hyponatremia

    C. Hypernatremia

    D. Hypercalcemia

    E. Hypokalemia

2. Which of the following statements is not true regarding rivastigmine?

   A. Gastrointestinal (GI) side effects with the transdermal formulation are lower compared with the oral formulation

   B. Following a break in therapy, retitration is recommended

   C. Concomitant anticholinergic agents can reduce rivastigmine efficacy

   D. The efficacy of the drug may diminish over time as the disease process advances

   E. It is an irreversible cholinesterase inhibitor

3. Lithium is efficacious for prophylaxis of bipolar affective illness in older patients. Given the physiologic changes associated with aging and medical comorbidities seen in the geriatric population, what is the recommended serum range for lithium during the maintenance phase of bipolar disorder in this age group to minimize the risk for drug toxicity?

   A. 0.4 to 0.8 mEq per L

   B. 0.6 to 1.2 mEq per L

   C. 0.2 to 0.6 mEq per L

   D. 1.0 to 1.2 mEq per L

   E. Any of the above

4. Which of the following is not recommended for the treatment of sundowning?

   A. Light therapy

   B. Benzodiazepines

   C. Structured activity program

   D. Antipsychotics

   E. Melatonin

5. Which of the following side effects associated with trazodone limits its usefulness in the management of behavioral problems in the geriatric population?

   A. Worsen cognition

   B. Excessive sedation

   C. Cardiac arrhythmias

   D. Orthostatic hypotension

   E. All of the above

6. All of the following physiologic changes in the elderly alter drug pharmacokinetics and increase the susceptibility to adverse effects of medications EXCEPT:

   A. Decreased glomerular filtration rate

   B. Decreased hepatic blood flow

   C. Reduced liver size

   D. Increased splanchnic blood flow

   E. Reduced first-pass metabolism

7. Which of the following acts as an antagonist at N-methyl-D-aspartate subtype of glutamate receptor?

   A. Topiramate

   B. Dextromethorphan

   C. Amantadine

   D. Memantine

   E. All of the above

8. Which of the following is true regarding memantine?

    A. No dose adjustments are required in renal or hepatic insufficiency

    B. Minimal risk for drug–drug interactions

    C. Combination therapy with acetylcholinesterase inhibitors does not offer added benefit

    D. It is U.S. Food and Drug Administration (FDA) approved for mild cognitive impairment (MCI)

    E. All of the above

9. A 65-year-old white man presents with depressive symptoms of 4-month duration. There are no psychotic features or evidence of dementia. You decide to prescribe a selective serotonin reuptake inhibitor (SSRI) to treat his depression. As you review his current medication list, the presence of which of the following herbal medication/micronutrients should alert you to the risk of bleeding when coadministered with SSRI?

    A. St. John's wort

    B. Valerian

    C. *Ginkgo biloba*

    D. Vitamin D

    E. All of the above

10. All of the following are potential side effects with donepezil therapy EXCEPT:

    A. Risk of GI bleeding

    B. Insomnia

    C. Nausea

    D. Diarrhea

    E. Loss of appetite

11. Which of the following statements regarding the safety of methylphenidate in the geriatric population is true?

    A. Increased risk of bleeding when coadministered with warfarin

    B. Can increase blood pressure

    C. Exacerbates tics

    D. Lead to anorexia

    E. All of the above

12. Methylphenidate is useful in the treatment of all the following geriatric conditions EXCEPT:

    A. Depressive symptoms in medically ill patients

    B. Augmentation of SSRIs in late-life depression

    C. Poststroke depression

    D. Apathy associated with dementia

    E. Depression associated with Parkinson disease

13. A 66-year-old African American man with HIV on protease inhibitors therapy presents with severe depressive and anxiety symptoms. You confirm a diagnosis of major depression and decide to start him on citalopram and alprazolam. As you order the medications, the pharmacy software alerts you to a potential drug–drug interaction between alprazolam and his protease inhibitors. Which of the following steps would have the greatest likelihood of minimizing the drug–drug interaction and ensuring therapeutic drug levels?

    A. Prescribe a lower than usual starting dose of alprazolam

    B. Prescribe a higher than usual starting dose of alprazolam

    C. Prescribe the usual starting dose of alprazolam

    D. Increase the dosage of his protease inhibitor and prescribe the usual starting dose of alprazolam

    E. Decrease the dosage of his protease inhibitor and prescribe the usual starting dose of alprazolam

14. There have been concerns about the widespread use of antipsychotics in nursing homes. Which of the following strategies is least beneficial in ensuring appropriate use of antipsychotics among nursing home patients with dementia-related behavioral problems?

A. Carefully documenting specific behaviors warranting antipsychotics

B. Ruling out preventable causes of disruptive behavior

C. Utilizing antipsychotics PRN orders instead of scheduled orders

D. Attempting dose reduction following stabilization of disruptive behavior

E. Close monitoring of antipsychotic adverse effects

15. Hospitalization among elderly patients is associated with a greater incidence of delirium. The Hospital Elder Life Program (HELP) is a new model of care designed to prevent functional and cognitive decline of older persons during hospitalization. The HELP found that lower rates of delirium were achieved in comparison with standard care when all the following risk factors were addressed EXCEPT:

A. Cognitive impairment

B. Immobility

C. Antipsychotic usage

D. Hearing impairment

E. Dehydration

16. Benzodiazepines are recommended to be used with caution in the elderly. Long-acting benzodiazepines can increase the risk of which of the following side effects in the elderly?

A. Hallucinations

B. Ataxia

C. Falls and hips fractures

D. Cognitive impairment

E. All of the above

17. Which of the following statements is true regarding the use of venlafaxine among elderly?

    A. Venlafaxine can be used as a first-line agent for the treatment of MDD

    B. Venlafaxine has significant drug–drug interactions with commonly used medications in elderly

    C. At moderate to higher doses, it inhibits the reuptake of serotonin

    D. Higher dosages of venlafaxine are needed to treat pain syndromes

    E. All of the above

18. Which of the statements is true regarding trazodone?

    A. It is a mixed serotonergic agonist–antagonist

    B. Its active metabolite, m-chlorophenylpiperazine (m-CPP), is a weak direct 5-Hydroxytryptamine (5-HT) agonist

    C. It is a potent blocker of presynaptic α_2-adrenergic receptors

    D. It is a weak blocker of postsynaptic α_1-adrenergic receptors

    E. It has moderate anticholinergic activity

19. Which of the following statements is not true regarding the use of lithium among elderly?

    A. Lithium levels should be maintained between 1 and 1.2 mEq per L

    B. They require lower dosage than younger patients to produce similar serum lithium levels

    C. Elderly are sensitive to neurologic side effects even at low doses

    D. Lithium is associated with delirium with serum levels as low as 1.5 mEq per L

    E. Aging increases the risk of lithium toxicity

20. SSRIs are shown to be efficacious in the treatment of which of the following symptoms among dementia patients?

    A. Agitation

    B. Disinhibition

    C. Delusions

    D. Hallucinations

    E. All of the above

21. Which of the following is true regarding the use of SSRIs in the elderly?

    A. It is recommended to start the SSRI at half their maximal efficacious dose

    B. Dosage is usually doubled after 3 to 4 weeks

    C. All the SSRIs are given in a single daily dose

    D. SSRIs should be used cautiously in patients taking nonsteroidal anti-inflammatory drugs (NSAIDs)

    E. All of the above

22. In which of the following coexisting conditions, SSRIs are not recommended for active and maintenance treatment of MDD?

    A. Cerebrovascular disease

    B. Cardiovascular disease

    C. MCI

    D. Dementia

    E. None of the above

23. Bupropion is used among the elderly for intolerance to SSRIs. Which of the following side effects would prompt switching to bupropion?

    A. Nausea

    B. Sexual side effects

    C. Severe fatigue

    D. Diarrhea

    E. All of the above

24. Which of the following is true regarding mirtazapine?

    A. It is a presynaptic α_2-receptor agonist

    B. Not associated with cognitive side effects

    C. Antinausea property is because of its inhibition at the 5-HT$_2$ and 5-HT$_3$ receptors

    D. Not associated with hematologic adverse effects

    E. All of the above

25. Bupropion's action on dopaminergic neurotransmission is associated with which of the following?

    A. Psychosis

    B. Gait disturbance

    C. Insomnia

    D. Agitation

    E. All of the above

26. SSRIs should be used with caution in which of the following elderly patients?

    A. Patients taking β-blockers

    B. Patients taking NSAIDs

    C. Patients taking low-dose aspirin

    D. Patients with hyponatremia

    E. All of the above

27. Mirtazapine is used among the elderly for intolerance to SSRIs. Which of the following side effects would prompt switching to mirtazapine?

    A. Nausea

    B. Sexual side effects

    C. Tremor

    D. Insomnia

    E. All of the above

28. Which of the following statements is true regarding the use of secondary amines tricyclic antidepressant (TCA) among the elderly?

    A. Secondary amines are not preferred because of their higher propensity to cause orthostasis and falls

    B. Secondary amines are preferred because of their linear pharmacokinetics

    C. Secondary amines are not preferred because of their anticholinergic effects

    D. TCAs are the first-line drugs in the treatment of late-life depression

    E. All of the above

29. Venlafaxine is known to cause which of the following cardiovascular side effect among the elderly?

    A. Dose-dependent hypertension

    B. Hypotension

    C. Arrhythmia

    D. Acute ischemia

    E. All of the above

30. Which of the following is true regarding cholinesterase inhibitors?

    A. Donepezil inhibits cholinesterase in the GI tract

    B. Galantamine has more peripheral activity than donepezil

    C. The primary mechanism of action of cholinesterase inhibitors is irreversible inhibition of acetylcholinesterase

    D. Galantamine may cause more sleeping difficulties than other cholinesterase inhibitors

    E. All of the above

31. Which of the following statements is not true regarding the antipsychotics use for the treatment of psychotic symptoms of any etiology in late life?

    A. Atypical antipsychotics have become first-line drugs

    B. Olanzapine is superior to promazine, haloperidol, and risperidone in efficacy and tolerability

    C. Olanzapine and risperidone have fewer severe extrapyramidal symptoms when compared with promazine and haloperidol

    D. Olanzapine causes more weight gain when compared with risperidone

    E. None of the above

32. Which of the following cholinesterase inhibitors is not FDA approved for the treatment of Alzheimer disease?

  A. Tacrine

  B. Donepezil

  C. Rivastigmine

  D. Galantamine

  E. None of the above

33. Valproic acid is used among the elderly with bipolar disorder who respond poorly to lithium. Which of the following symptoms would prompt switching to valproic acid?

  A. Bipolar patients with prominent dysphoria

  B. Rapid cycling

  C. Mania associated with dementia

  D. Secondary mania

  E. All of the above

34. Older patients taking carbamazepine are at higher risk for developing which of the following?

  A. Drug-induced leucopenia

  B. Drug-induced agranulocytosis

  C. Ataxia

  D. Drug interactions

  E. All of the above

35. A 72-year-old man with Parkinson disease was brought in by his son for depressive symptoms. He scored 9 on the Geriatric Depression Scale and 27 out of 30 on the Montreal Cognitive Assessment (MOCA). He stopped taking L-dopa because of adverse effects. He was on fluoxetine 20 mg for 4 months but discontinued it because of worsening movement disorder. Currently he is not on any antidepressant. His blood workup and urine analysis are within normal limits. Which of the following would be a reasonable treatment choice?

    A. Galantamine

    B. Rivastigmine

    C. Pramipexole

    D. Fluoxetine

    E. All of the above

36. Atypical antipsychotics increase the risk of which of the following?

    A. Type 2 diabetes mellitus

    B. Cardiovascular effects

    C. Sudden death in elderly

    D. Cerebrovascular effects

    E. All of the above

37. A 74-year-old man with Alzheimer dementia presents to you for medication management. You decide to start rivastigmine and adhere to the prescribed dosing schedule by starting him on 1.5 mg twice a day. After 2 weeks, you decide to increase the dose to 3 mg twice a day. The patient experiences nausea and vomiting within 3 days of increasing the dose. On examination, his vital signs are stable. What should be the next best step?

    A. Change the dosing schedule to 1.5 mg twice a day

    B. Discontinue treatment for several doses and then restart at a lower dose

    C. Continue the same dose (3 mg twice a day) and reevaluate in a week

    D. Prescribe promethazine while maintaining the dose of rivastigmine at 3 mg twice a day

    E. Order barium swallow

38. A 68-year-old man with Alzheimer dementia with end-stage renal disease presents to you for medication management. He is on dialysis and on a waiting list for kidney transplant. Which of the following cholinesterase inhibitor is not recommended for this patient?

    A. Donepezil

    B. Galantamine

    C. Rivastigmine

    D. Tacrine

    E. None of the above

39. Which of the following classes of medications is efficacious and safe in the management of chronic agitation associated with dementia?

    A. β-Blockers

    B. Benzodiazepines

    C. Atypical antipsychotics

    D. SSRIs

    E. All of the above

40. Which of the following is true regarding the management of dementia?

    A. Donepezil is FDA approved for mild, moderate, and severe Alzheimer disease

    B. Galantamine is FDA approved for mild to moderate Alzheimer disease

    C. Rivastigmine is FDA approved for mild to moderate Alzheimer disease

    D. Memantine is FDA approved for moderate to severe Alzheimer disease

    E. All of the above

41. Despite a half-life of 1 hour, the cholinesterase inhibitor rivastigmine is dosed twice a day. Which of the following statements is the best explanation for this?

    A. More frequent dosing of rivastigmine can cause intolerable GI side effects

    B. Rivastigmine remains bound to cholinesterase, thus remaining therapeutically active for 10 hours

    C. Rivastigmine remains bound at the nicotinic receptor site, thus remaining therapeutically active for 10 hours

    D. Frequent dosing helps to control the behavioral disturbances

    E. All of the above

42. Which of the following is true regarding the treatment of Parkinson disease dementia (PDD)?

    A. Anticholinergic medication are the treatment of choice

    B. Rivastigmine is the only FDA-approved treatment for PDD

    C. Treat with the maximum tolerated dose of dopamine agonist

    D. Clozapine is FDA approved for behavioral disturbances associated with PDD

    E. All of the above

43. A 66-year-old Caucasian man on warfarin therapy for atrial fibrillation is presenting with depressed mood, poor energy levels, and sleeping difficulties. He has a past psychiatric history significant for major depression. He does not remember his past psychotropic trials. Which of the following is true regarding coadministration of SSRI with warfarin?

A. Increase in prothrombin time is reported with fluvoxamine and fluoxetine when combined with warfarin

B. Competitive inhibition of CYP2C9 could result in potentiation of warfarin-induced anticoagulation when coadministered with SSRI

C. SSRIs increase the risk of bleeding by altering platelet aggregation, and the risk of bleeding may be further increased when combined with warfarin

D. Fluoxetine, fluvoxamine, and paroxetine appear to have the highest potential for CYP2C9 inhibition

E. All of the above

44. Which of the following cholinesterase inhibitors is rarely used in view of its several side effects, mainly hepatic toxicity?

A. Galantamine

B. Rivastigmine

C. Tacrine

D. Donepezil

E. Memantine

45. Atypical antipsychotic medications are frequently used to treat Alzheimer patients with delusions, aggression, and hallucinations. Which of the following statements regarding the outcomes of the National Institutes of Health (NIH)-funded Clinical Antipsychotic Trial of Intervention Effectiveness study for Alzheimer Disease (CATIE-AD) is/are true?

    A. In CATIE-AD, atypical antipsychotics were associated with worsening cognitive functioning compared with placebo

    B. There were no significant differences on measures of effectiveness between the atypical antipsychotics and placebo

    C. CATIE-AD results indicate that patients may benefit symptomatically from treatment with atypical antipsychotics; however, the medications had little effect on measures of functional abilities, quality of life, or caregiving time needed

    D. One of the advantages of the CATIE-AD trial is that it included outpatients in usual care settings

    E. All of the above

46. Antipsychotics use among the elderly has a black box warning for increased risk of mortality from which of the following?

    A. Cardiovascular

    B. Cereberovascular

    C. Endocrine

    D. Respiratory system

    E. Musculoskeletal

47. All of the following are true of the rivastigmine transdermal system (Exelon Patch) EXCEPT:

    A. The patch should be changed every 24 hours

    B. A patient who is on a total daily dose of 6 to 12 mg of oral rivastigmine may be directly switched to Exelon Patch 9.5 mg per 24 hours

    C. Dose increases should occur only after a minimum of 2 weeks at the previous dose

    D. Dose increases should occur only after the previous dose was well tolerated

    E. None of the above

48. An 80-year-old Caucasian man was brought to your clinic by his son who raised concerns that his dad stopped caring for himself. He is usually a clean and active person, and it is surprising to see him unshaven. On further questioning, the patient denied any depression. Geriatric Depression Scale score was 2. He scored 22 out of 30 on MOCA. He was diagnosed with Alzheimer dementia and is currently on Donepezil 5 mg QHS. He has prominent apathy. Which of the following would be an appropriate treatment for his apathy?

    A. Fluoxetine

    B. Bupropion

    C. Methylphenidate

    D. Aripiprazole

    E. Desipramine

Answers

1. **Answer: B.** Hyponatremia

SSRIs therapy has been associated with hyponatremia (serum sodium concentration <130 mEq per L). The incidence of this dangerous side effect with SSRIs ranges from 0.5% to 32%. Elderly patients are more prone to SSRI-induced hyponatremia. The precise mechanism by which SSRIs cause hyponatremia is unknown; however, it is believed that it may be because of development of the syndrome of inappropriate secretion of antidiuretic hormone (SIADH).

2. **Answer: E.** It is an irreversible cholinesterase inhibitor

Rivastigmine is a reversible acetylcholinesterase inhibitor approved for the treatment of Alzheimer disease. Rivastigmine is unique in that it inhibits both butyrylcholinesterase and acetylcholinesterase. Rapid dose titration increases the incidence of GI side effects. Rivastigmine transdermal system offers benefits for patients who have trouble swallowing pills and is associated with lower incidence nausea and vomiting. As the Alzheimer disease process advances, there are fewer functional cholinergic neurons that might explain the gradual loss of therapeutic benefit with the drug.

3. **Answer: A.** 0.4 to 0.8 mEq per L

Elderly patients often require lower lithium dosages to achieve therapeutic serum levels. They may also exhibit adverse reactions at serum levels ordinarily tolerated by younger patients. In addition, medical conditions leading to volume depletion, to the use of NSAIDs, and to the use of thiazide diuretics can increase lithium levels in the older population. A serum lithium level between 0.4 and 0.8 mEq per L is considered safe and therapeutic. More frequent monitoring of serum lithium levels is required in elderly patients.

4. **Answer: B.** Benzodiazepines

Management of sundowning includes both pharmacologic and nonpharmacologic approaches. Light therapy (keeping lights on into the hours of darkness), elimination of taking away of daytime naps, sleep hygiene, and structured activity are recommended. Medications useful in sundowning include melatonin and atypical antipsychotics. Antipsychotics agents should be limited for short-term use because there is an increased mortality risk in elderly patients with dementia. Benzodiazepines are ineffective and can in fact worsen symptoms of sundowning.

5. **Answer: E.** All of the above

Trazodone causes orthostatic hypotension because of α_1-adrenergic receptor blockade. Cardiac arrhythmias and syncope have been reported with trazodone. Elderly patients may be more sensitive to the sedating property of trazodone. Finally, there have been reports of trazodone causing memory impairment.

6. **Answer: D.** Increased splanchnic blood flow

Physiologic changes associated with aging can alter drug pharmacokinetics and pharmacodynamics. Aging is also associated with reduced liver mass and decreased hepatic blood flow resulting in decreased hepatic clearance and first-pass metabolism. However, splanchnic blood flow decreases with aging, which reduces drug absorption.

7. **Answer: E.** All of the above

Topiramate, dextromethorphan, amantadine, and memantine have antagonistic properties at N-methyl-D-aspartate subtype of glutamate receptor. In addition, topiramate blocks sodium channels, dextromethorphan acts as a σ_1-receptor agonist, and amantadine possesses antiviral and anticholinergic effects.

8. **Answer: B.** Minimal risk for drug–drug interactions

Memantine is eliminated by kidneys, and dose reduction is recommended in renal insufficiency. It minimally inhibits cytochrome P450 enzymes. Currently, there are no FDA-approved drugs for MCI.

9. **Answer: C.** *Ginkgo biloba*

There have been reports of spontaneous bleeding associated with *G. biloba*. This risk is higher when coadministered with SSRIs that have known bleeding tendencies. St. John's wort may cause serotonin syndrome when coadministered with SSRIs. Valerian is used for insomnia and anxiety, and it causes minimal adverse effects.

10. **Answer: A.** Risk of GI bleeding

Loss of appetite, weight loss, nausea, vomiting, and diarrhea are common side effects of donepezil. Most of these side effects are because of central and peripheral inhibition of acetylcholinesterase.

11. **Answer: E.** All of the above

Methylphenidate and other psychostimulants can exacerbate tics, anorexia, and hypertension. Methylphenidate may inhibit the metabolism of coumarin anticoagulants leading to increased risk of bleeding.

12. **Answer: E.** Depression associated with Parkinson disease

There are no significant data to support the use of methylphenidate in depression associated with Parkinson disease.

13. **Answer: A.** Prescribe a lower than usual starting dose of alprazolam

Protease inhibitors are metabolized primarily by cytochrome isoenzyme P450 3A (CYP3A). All protease inhibitors increase psychotropic drug concentrations if the major route of metabolism of the psychotropic drug is the CYP3A system. Alprazolam concentrations may be increased, and dosage reductions may be needed to prevent oversedation.

14. **Answer: C.** Utilizing antipsychotics PRN orders instead of scheduled orders

PRN use of antipsychotic in nursing homes is discouraged except in situations in which antipsychotics doses are being titrated upward or downward or when the patient is in imminent danger of harming self or others.

15. **Answer: C.** Antipsychotic usage

The HELP, developed by Yale University and now adopted by several hospitals, found that lower rates of delirium were achieved in comparison with standard care when the following risk factors were addressed — cognitive impairment, immobility, visual impairment, hearing impairment, and dehydration. Antipsychotics have no role in the prevention of delirium.

16. **Answer: E.** All of the above

Long half-life benzodiazepines are usually not recommended for the elderly patient because they are more likely to accumulate and not rapidly eliminated. Long half-life benzodiazepines may increase the risk of daytime sedation, lethargy, cognitive impairment, falls, ataxia, and hallucinations. Elderly patients are more prone to these side effects given their pharmacodynamic sensitivity to central nervous system (CNS) acting drugs and reduced clearance because of hepatic compromise.

17. **Answer: D.** Higher dosages are needed to treat pain syndromes

Venlafaxine is not recommended as a first-line agent in the elderly. It is reserved for people who do not respond to SSRI. Venlafaxine does not inhibit any of the major cytochrome P450 isoenzymes to cause clinically significant drug–drug interactions. It inhibits the reuptake of serotonin even at low doses. Venlafaxine at its minimal effective dose, 75 mg per day, acts as a selective 5-HT reuptake inhibitor, whereas at higher doses, such as 225 and 375 mg per day, acts as a dual 5-HT and norepinephrine reuptake inhibitor. Higher dosages (i.e., 225 mg per day or more) are usually needed to treat pain syndromes because venlafaxine's antinociceptive effects are mediated by its action at α_2-adrenergic receptors.

18. **Answer: A.** It is a mixed serotonergic agonist–antagonist

Trazodone is a mixed serotonergic agonist–antagonist. Its active metabolite, m-CPP, is a potent direct 5-HT agonist. Trazodone is a relatively weak blocker of presynaptic α_2-adrenergic receptors and a relatively potent antagonist of postsynaptic α_1-adrenergic receptors. It lacks anticholinergic side effects and is especially useful in patients with prostatic hypertrophy, closed-angle glaucoma, or severe constipation.

19. **Answer: A.** Lithium levels should be maintained between 1 and 1.2 mEq per L

Lithium levels should be kept as low as 0.4 to 0.8 mEq per L in elderly because they are more sensitive to neurologic side effects even at lower lithium levels. Delirium can occur with serum levels of 1.5 mEq per L because of lithium's anticholinergic activity.

20. **Answer: E.** All of the above

Randomized- and placebo-controlled trials have shown that SSRIs may be efficacious in the treatment of behavioral disturbances associated not only with dementia such as agitation and disinhibition but also with the psychotic symptoms such as hallucinations and delusions.

21. **Answer: D.** SSRIs should be used cautiously in patients taking NSAIDs

Usual starting dose of SSRIs is half the minimal efficacious dose. It is usually doubled after 1 week. All the SSRIs can be given in a single daily dose except for fluvoxamine, which is administered in two divided doses. SSRIs may cause platelet activation and act synergistically with NSAIDs and low-dose aspirin in increasing the risk of GI bleeding.

22. **Answer: E.** None of the above

SSRIs are safe and are well tolerated among the elderly with conditions such as schizophrenia, MDD, MCI, dementia, cerebrovascular, and cardiovascular disease.

23. **Answer: E.** All of the above

Bupropion is used among the elderly when they experience side effects such as nausea, sexual side effects, fatigue, and diarrhea while using SSRIs.

24. **Answer: C.** Antinausea property is because of its inhibition at the 5-HT_2 and 5-HT_3 receptors

Mirtazapine is a presynaptic α_2-receptor antagonist. Cognitive deficits are seen with mirtazapine use because of its antihistaminergic and sedative effects. It is known to impair driving and has been associated with delirium as well. Hematologic adverse effects such as neutropenia and agranulocytosis have been reported with its use.

25. **Answer: E.** All of the above

Psychosis, gait disturbance, falls, hip fractures, insomnia, and agitation can be associated with bupropion's action on dopaminergic neurotransmission.

26. **Answer: E.** All of the above

SSRIs are associated with bradycardia. SSRIs may cause platelet activation and act synergistically with NSAIDs and low-dose aspirin in increasing the risk of GI bleeding. Syndrome of SIADH is a dangerous adverse effect of SSRI. Hence, it should not be used in the elderly when they have already had hyponatremia.

27. **Answer: E.** All of the above

Mirtazapine is used among the elderly when they experience side effects such as nausea, sexual side effects, tremor, or insomnia.

28. **Answer: B.** Secondary amines are preferred because of their linear pharmacokinetics

TCAs are the third-line drugs in the treatment of late-life depression because of their adverse effects. Secondary amines such as desipramine and nortriptyline are preferred among the TCAs because of their lower propensity to cause orthostasis and falls, their linear pharmacokinetics, and their modest anticholinergic effects. The linear kinetics of secondary amines means that if the dose is increased, the plasma concentration will be increased proportionally.

29. **Answer: E.** All of the above

Venlafaxine is known to cause dose-dependent hypertension, hypotension, arrhythmia, or acute ischemia.

30. **Answer: B.** Galantamine has more peripheral activity than donepezil

Donepezil selectively inhibits cholinesterase in the CNS with little peripheral activity in the GI tract, whereas galantamine has more peripheral activity. The primary mechanism of action of cholinesterase inhibitors is reversible, inhibition of acetylcholinesterase. Donepezil may cause more sleeping difficulties than other cholinesterase inhibitors.

31. **Answer: B.** Olanzapine is superior to promazine, haloperidol, and risperidone in efficacy and tolerability

Both olanzapine and risperidone have superior efficacy and tolerability to promazine and haloperidol.

32. **Answer: E.** None of the above

Tacrine, donepezil, rivastigmine, and galantamine are all approved by FDA for the treatment of Alzheimer disease. However, the use of tacrine is not recommended because of its potential hepatotoxic effects.

33. **Answer: E.** All of the above

Bipolar patients with prominent dysphoria or rapid cycling with poor response to lithium do well with anticonvulsants such as valproic acid. Mania associated with dementia may respond better to anticonvulsants.

34. **Answer: E.** All of the above

Older patients on carbamazepine are at higher risk for drug-induced leucopenia, drug-induced agranulocytosis, ataxia, and drug interactions.

35. Answer: C. Pramipexole

Recent studies indicate that pramipexole, a D3 dopamine agonist, is efficacious in improving depressive symptoms in Parkinson disease and was significantly superior to placebo. Double-blind, placebo-controlled studies report that nortriptyline and desipramine were superior to placebo and SSRIs. Rivastigmine is approved for PDD and not for depression in Parkinson disease.

36. Answer: E. All of the above

Atypical antipsychotics are not approved for dementia-related psychosis because they are reported to increase the risk of cerebrovascular events and sudden death. They also increase the risk of cardiovascular effects and type 2 diabetes mellitus.

37. Answer: B. Discontinue treatment for several doses and then restart at a lower dose

Incidence of nausea and vomiting is much higher with initial titration of rivastigmine. It is recommended to discontinue treatment for several doses and then restart at a lower dose rather than to changing/lowering the dosing schedule. There is no evidence of esophageal rupture, which may occur with severe vomiting; hence, there is no need for further investigations such as barium swallow.

38. Answer: C. Rivastigmine

Rivastigmine's metabolism is affected by renal function, and therefore, it is not recommended for patients with renal insufficiency.

39. Answer: D. SSRIs

SSRIs are safe and efficacious in the management of chronic agitation associated with dementia.

40. Answer: E. All of the above

Donepezil is FDA approved for mild, moderate, and severe Alzheimer disease. Galantamine and rivastigmine are FDA approved for mild to moderate Alzheimer disease. Memantine is FDA approved for moderate to severe Alzheimer disease.

41. **Answer: B.** Rivastigmine remains bound to cholinesterase, thus remaining therapeutically active for 10 hours

Despite a half-life of 1 hour, rivastigmine is dosed twice a day because it remains bound to cholinesterases, thus remaining therapeutically active for 10 hours. It is a nicotinic allosteric modulator, but it does not remain bound at the nicotinic receptor site. Frequent dosing does not help to control the behavioral disturbances.

42. **Answer: B.** Rivastigmine is the only FDA-approved treatment for PDD

Current treatment recommendation for PDD is to discontinue or avoid anticholinergic medication in view of developing delirium. Among elderly, reduce the dose of dopamine agonist and treat with the minimum tolerated dose. Behavioral disturbances or psychosis associated with PDD may be treated with quetiapine or clozapine because they have lower extrapyramidal side effects (EPSE). However, these agents are not approved by FDA.

43. **Answer: E.** All of the above

SSRIs are known for the risk of bleeding, and, when coadministered with warfarin, the risk is increased further. Besides this pharmacodynamic interaction, it is postulated that SSRIs competitively inhibit CYP2C9 resulting in potentiation of warfarin-induced anticoagulation. Among the SSRIs, fluoxetine, fluvoxamine, and paroxetine appear to have the highest potential for CYP2C9 inhibition.

44. **Answer: C.** Tacrine

Within 6 to 8 weeks of initiation of tacrine, dose-related elevations of aspartate amino transaminase and alkaline phosphatase are seen in 20% to 40% of Alzheimer patients. Hepatotoxicity, liver failure, jaundice, and hepatitis that limit its use in the management of Alzheimer dementia have also been reported.

45. **Answer: E.** All of the above

The NIH-funded CATIE-AD enrolled 421 participants nationwide with Alzheimer dementia and delusions, aggression, hallucinations, or agitation. The study investigators determined medications' effectiveness by balancing their associated benefits with their associated risks. There were no significant differences in measures of effectiveness between the atypical antipsychotics and placebo. The antipsychotic medications were associated with a greater burden of side effects. The atypical antipsychotics also worsened cognitive functioning at a magnitude consistent with 1 year of deterioration compared with placebo.

46. **Answer: A.** Cardiovascular

Studies report that the rate of death in antipsychotics-treated patients was about 4.5%, when compared with 2.6% in the placebo group. Among variety of causes that caused the deaths, most were either cardiovascular such as heart failure and sudden death or infectious in nature such as pneumonia.

47. **Answer: C.** Dose increases should occur only after a minimum of 2 weeks at the previous dose

Rivastigmine transdermal system (Exelon Patch) should be changed every 24 hours. Patients on a total daily dose of 6 to 12 mg of oral rivastigmine may be directly switched to Exelon Patch 9.5 mg per 24 hours, and those receiving <6 mg per day can switch to 4.6 mg per 24 hours. Dose increases should occur only after a minimum of 4 weeks at the previous dose and after the previous dose was well tolerated.

48. **Answer: C.** Methylphenidate

Methylphenidate has good evidence in managing patients with apathy.

Chapter 4

Addiction Psychopharmacology

Questions

1. Which of the following statements regarding naltrexone is true?

   A. Naltrexone is a strong antagonist at δ- and κ-type opioid receptors

   B. Naltrexone's antagonistic effect on μ-type opioid receptors is responsible for causing nausea

   C. Naltrexone has >90% oral bioavailability

   D. Naltrexone undergoes extensive first-pass metabolism

   E. All of the above

2. Which of the following statements is true regarding varenicline?

   A. Varenicline's antagonistic activity at a subtype of the nicotinic receptor is responsible for its mechanism of action

   B. It is efficacious in relapse prevention

   C. Food has no effect on its bioavailability

   D. Patients quit successfully with bupropion than with varenicline

   E. Diarrhea is the most common side effect

3. Buprenorphine's advantages over clonidine, in the management of patients with opioid withdrawal, include better control of which of the following symptoms?

    A. Nausea

    B. Cramping

    C. Craving

    D. Diarrhea

    E. Sweating

4. All of the following are true regarding buprenorphine induction EXCEPT:

    A. It is recommended that patients present in mild, observable, spontaneous opioid withdrawal on the day of buprenorphine induction

    B. Patients are expected to spend at least 2 hours in the office during the induction day

    C. The maximum buprenorphine dose recommended for the first day is 6 mg

    D. Because buprenorphine is a partial opioid agonist, it is possible that the drug may precipitate opioid withdrawal

    E. For induction, only the sublingual buprenorphine formulation and not the transdermal formulation should be used

5. Which of the following statements regarding buprenorphine is true?

    A. Buprenorphine is given sublingually and not orally to minimize abuse

    B. Buprenorphine prolongs the QTc interval at therapeutic doses

    C. Buprenorphine has a slow rate of dissociation from opioid receptors

    D. Buprenorphine is a partial agonist at the κ-opioid receptors and an antagonist at μ-opioid receptors

    E. All of the above

6. All of the following statements regarding naltrexone are true EXCEPT:

   A. It is a competitive antagonist at the opioid receptor

   B. The drug acts by reducing the rewarding effects of alcohol through blocking the release of dopamine

   C. Concurrent use of tramadol, a centrally acting opioid analgesic, with naltrexone can precipitate acute opiate withdrawal reaction

   D. A long-acting injectable preparation of naltrexone is available

   E. It is Food and Drug Administration (FDA) approved for opiate and alcohol dependence

7. What is the minimum washout period for patients taking methadone before the first dose of an opioid receptor antagonist such as naloxone or naltrexone?

   A. 5 days

   B. 2 weeks

   C. 10 days

   D. 3 weeks

   E. 4 weeks

8. A 27-year-old white man was diagnosed with brief psychotic disorder. After 6 months, he started drinking alcohol heavily and was given a diagnosis of alcohol dependence. His family threatened to disown him, following which he agreed for an admission to a chemical dependency unit. He actively participated in group therapy and individual therapy but refused medications. With persuasion, he was commenced on disulfiram as an aversive conditioning treatment for alcohol dependence. Soon after his discharge, he started acting strangely; he believes that the FDA is after him and refuses to leave his house for fear of being monitored by aliens. Physical examination is unremarkable. Drug testing is negative, and he denies relapse. What is the most likely diagnosis?

   A. Substance-induced mood disorder

   B. Disulfiram-induced exacerbation of psychosis

   C. Schizophrenia

   D. Schizophreniform disorder

   E. Delirium tremens

9. All of the following medications are FDA approved for the treatment of smoking cessation pharmacotherapy EXCEPT:

    A. Varenicline

    B. Bupropion

    C. Nicotine

    D. Clonidine

    E. None of the above

10. All of the following statements regarding methadone are true EXCEPT:

    A. FDA indicated for the management of opioid abuse and moderate to severe pain

    B. Contraindicated in patients with acute bronchial asthma

    C. Major route of methadone metabolism is through Cytochrome P450 3A4 (CYP3A4)

    D. Starting doses of methadone can be as high as 80 to 100 mg per day

    E. None of the above

11. In addition to its role in alcohol dependence, disulfiram is clinically useful in which of the following substance dependence disorders?

    A. Methamphetamine dependence

    B. Marijuana dependence

    C. Cocaine dependence

    D. Nicotine dependence

    E. Inhalant dependence in adolescents

12. All of the following opioid antagonists are indicated in the management of opioid overdose EXCEPT:

    A. Naloxone

    B. Naltrexone

    C. Nalmefene

    D. Nalbuphine

    E. None of the above

13. Which of the following agents has no role in the management of alcohol withdrawal syndrome?

    A. Carbamazepine

    B. Chlordiazepoxide

    C. Lorazepam

    D. Diazepam

    E. None of the above

14. All of the following are therapeutic uses of clonidine EXCEPT:

    A. Opioid withdrawal

    B. Nicotine withdrawal

    C. Stimulant withdrawal

    D. Alcohol withdrawal

    E. Benzodiazepine withdrawal

15. All of the following are differences between illicit γ-hydroxybutyrate (GHB) and sodium oxybate EXCEPT:

    A. Illicit GHB is taken at frequent intervals, whereas sodium oxybate is taken at bedtime

    B. Illicit GHB is often taken with other illicit drugs, whereas sodium oxybate is not to be taken with alcohol or central nervous system (CNS) depressants

    C. Illicit GHB is more widely available than sodium oxybate

    D. GHB for nonmedical use is schedule III drug, and when prescribed for medical indications, it is a schedule I substance

    E. None of the above

16. A 21-year-old male college student was brought in to the emergency department by his roommate for agitation and bizarre behavior for the past 2 hours. His roommate reports that the patient returned from a party and used a white crystalline powder. During examination, the patient appears confused and cannot engage in a conversation. He smells of alcohol, and his physical examination is remarkable for tachycardia, nystagmus, and miosis. Besides routine investigations and supportive care, which of the following might have a role in elimination of the drug from the patient's body?

    A. Alkalization of urine

    B. Acidification of urine

    C. Administration of phenobarbital

    D. Administration of lidocaine

    E. All of the above

17. A 43-year-old Caucasian man with alcohol-induced cirrhosis of liver was admitted for upper gastrointestinal (GI) bleed. His variceal bleeding was treated during this admission. He is medically stable and ready for discharge. He is requesting medications to help him prevent relapsing on alcohol. Which of the following would be your best choice?

   A. Naltrexone

   B. Lorazepam

   C. Disulfiram

   D. Acamprosate

   E. All of the above

18. Which of the following antidepressants can be considered as a second-line therapy for smoking cessation?

   A. Nortriptyline

   B. Mirtazapine

   C. Venlafaxine

   D. Duloxetine

   E. Fluoxetine

19. Which of the following nicotine-replacement formulations produces the most rapid rise in nicotine levels?

   A. Nicotine vapor inhalers

   B. Nicotine nasal spray

   C. Nicotine lozenges

   D. Nicotine gum

   E. Nicotine transdermal patch

20. All of the following statements regarding methadone are true EXCEPT:

    A. Concurrent use of methadone and ziprasidone can increase QTc interval

    B. Mean plasma half-life of methadone is about 24 hours

    C. Methadone induces its own metabolism and can increase its clearance

    D. Methadone has very low risk for abuse

    E. Methadone is an agonist at the μ-opiate receptor

21. The unpleasant disulfiram-alcohol reaction is caused by accumulation of which of the following?

    A. Acetyl coenzyme A

    B. Acetaldehyde

    C. Aldehyde dehydrogenase

    D. Pyruvate

    E. Malondialdehyde

22. All of the following statements about acamprosate are true EXCEPT:

    A. Acamprosate attenuates hyperglutamatergic states that occur during early abstinence

    B. Acamprosate should be initiated in patients who are abstinent at treatment

    C. Like naltrexone, acamprosate has shown to specially reduce heavy drinking

    D. The FDA-recommended dose of acamprosate is 660 mg twice a day

    E. It is contraindicated in severe renal impairment

23. Naltrexone should not be prescribed concurrently with which of the following?

    A. Tramadol

    B. Oxycodone

    C. Diazepam

    D. Fluoxetine

    E. Diclofenac sodium

24. The efficacy of bupropion in tobacco cessation is because of which of the following?

    A. Antagonizing nicotinic acetylcholine receptors

    B. Dopamine reuptake inhibition

    C. Noradrenaline reuptake inhibitor

    D. Attenuate nicotine withdrawal symptoms

    E. All of the above

25. A 36-year-old African American man is admitted to the intensive care unit for management of alcohol intoxication. His past medical history includes gastroesophageal reflux disease (GERD), cirrhosis of liver, and hypertension. There is documentation of delirium tremens in his chart. His initial blood alcohol level is 350. A repeat blood alcohol level in 6 hours comes back as 75. Which of the following would be the most appropriate drug in his management?

    A. Chlordiazepoxide

    B. Lorazepam

    C. Diazepam

    D. Carbamazepine

    E. Clonidine

26. Which of the following agents is the treatment of choice for opiate overdose?

    A. Buprenorphine

    B. Methadone

    C. Flumazenil

    D. Naloxone

    E. Phentolamine

27. A 37-year-old African American man was admitted to the hospital for his elective septoplasty. He has alcohol dependence and is currently taking naltrexone. You are consulted regarding his pain management and clearance for surgery. What is your next best step?

    A. Initiate hydrocodone therapy

    B. Immediate surgery with diclofenac sodium for pain control

    C. Emergency surgery with hydrocodone for pain control

    D. Stop naltrexone and plan for surgery within 24 hours

    E. Stop naltrexone and plan for surgery in 72 hours

28. A patient with alcohol dependence and generalized anxiety disorder is requesting a medication for use on an as-needed basis for his anxiety attacks. Which of the following medications would be the most appropriate choice?

    A. Paroxetine

    B. Hydroxyzine

    C. Buspirone

    D. Lorazepam

    E. Chlordiazepoxide

29. Disulfiram should not be prescribed concurrently with which of the following?

    A. Fluoxetine

    B. Tramadol

    C. Naltrexone

    D. Metronidazole

    E. Lorazepam

30. Which of the following must be closely monitored during naltrexone therapy?

    A. Liver function test (LFT)

    B. Renal function test

    C. Thyroid profile

    D. Lipid panel

    E. Platelet count

Answers

1. **Answer: E.** All the above

Naltrexone is a strong antagonist at δ- and κ-type opioid receptors. Its antagonistic effect on μ-type opioid receptors is responsible for causing nausea. Naltrexone is rapidly well absorbed with approximately 96% of the dose absorbed from the GI tract; however, it is subject to significant first-pass metabolism.

2. **Answer: C.** Food has no effect on its bioavailability

Varenicline is a partial agonist–antagonist at $\alpha_4\beta_2$ subtype of the nicotinic acetylcholine receptors. Varenicline works by blocking nicotine from attaching to the receptors and decreases the release of dopamine. A recent meta-analysis reported that more participants quit successfully with varenicline than with bupropion. The effectiveness of varenicline as an aid to relapse prevention has not been clearly established. Vomiting is the most common side effect of varenicline. It does not cause diarrhea but causes constipation.

3. **Answer: A.** Nausea

Although clonidine reduces many of the autonomic effects of opioid withdrawal syndrome, nausea is better controlled with buprenorphine.

4. **Answer: C.** The maximum buprenorphine dose recommended for the first day is 6 mg

Buprenorphine is a partial opioid agonist; it is possible that the drug may precipitate opioid withdrawal. Thus, it is recommended that on the day of buprenorphine induction patients present with mild, observable spontaneous opioid withdrawal on the day of buprenorphine induction. Patients are expected to spend at least 2 hours in the office during the induction day. The recommended maximum dose of buprenorphine on the first day is 12 to 16 mg. Subsequently buprenorphine dose can be titrated and maximum daily dose is about 24 mg per day. For induction, only the sublingual buprenorphine formulation and not the transdermal formulation should be used.

5. **Answer: C.** Buprenorphine has a slow rate of dissociation from opioid receptors

When buprenorphine is administered orally, it is extensively metabolized by liver and intestines resulting in very low bioavailability. Buprenorphine can prolong the QTc interval at higher doses, and there are no reports of clinically significant QTc elevation at therapeutic doses. Buprenorphine has a slow rate of dissociation from opioid receptors, and, when terminated after chronic therapy, no withdrawal syndrome is observed. It is a partial μ-opioid receptor agonist and an antagonist at κ-opioid receptor.

6. **Answer: C.** Concurrent use of tramadol, a centrally acting opioid analgesic, with naltrexone can precipitate acute opiate withdrawal reaction

Naltrexone produces antagonistic effects by competitively displacing opiate molecules at opiate receptors as well as blocking the access of narcotics to opiate receptor sites. Concurrent administration of naltrexone and opioid analgesics is contraindicated because naltrexone will reverse the effects of narcotic analgesics resulting in acute withdrawal symptoms. Although tramadol is a centrally acting opioid analgesic that exerts its effect by binding to μ-opioid receptors, there is no drug–drug interaction between naltrexone and tramadol. Hence, tramadol can be safely used for analgesia in patients on naltrexone therapy. Naltrexone is a competitive antagonist at the opioid receptor and FDA approved for opiate and alcohol dependence. It acts by reducing the rewarding effects of alcohol through blocking the release of dopamine. A long-acting injectable preparation of naltrexone is available.

7. **Answer: C.** 10 days

Patients receiving naltrexone for narcotic addiction should be detoxified before naltrexone administration because naltrexone will reverse the effects of narcotic analgesics in dependent persons, resulting in withdrawal symptoms within 5 minutes of ingestion. Patients on methadone should be opioid free for a minimum of 7 to 10 days before initiating treatment with naltrexone.

8. **Answer: B.** Disulfiram-induced exacerbation of psychosis

Disulfiram is associated with wide ranges of psychiatric effects such as depression, agitation, paranoia, and bizarre behaviors. Disulfiram use is contraindicated in psychoses. The emergence of psychotic symptoms with the patient's treatment with disulfiram suggests that disulfiram contributed to the occurrence of his symptoms. His presentation is inconsistent with the other listed choices.

9. **Answer: D.** Clonidine

Varenicline, nicotine replacement therapy, and bupropion are FDA-approved treatments for nicotine dependence.

10. **Answer: D.** Starting doses of methadone can be as high as 80 to 100 mg per day

Major route of methadone metabolism is through CYP3A4. Maximum daily dose of methadone can be as high as 80 to 100 mg per day, not the starting dose. Methadone is FDA indicated in the treatment of the management of opioid abuse and moderate to severe pain. Methadone is known to cause respiratory depression. It is contraindicated in patients with asthma and should be used with extreme caution in patients with decreased respiratory reserve such as asthma, chronic obstructive pulmonary disease, severe obesity, and sleep apnea.

11. **Answer: C.** Cocaine dependence

There is no FDA-approved treatment for cocaine dependence. There are some data from studies supporting the clinical use of disulfiram for the treatment of cocaine dependence. Disulfiram is an inhibitor of aldehyde dehydrogenase, which is directly relevant to its role in curbing alcohol consumption. However, disulfiram also inhibits dopamine β-hydroxylase, which catalyzes the conversion of dopamine to norepinephrine and thereby controls the norepinephrine-to-dopamine ratio in the CNS. Because dopamine mediates the drug seeking and reward behavior in cocaine dependence, this effect of disulfiram on dopamine neurotransmission is postulated to explain its role in decreasing cocaine cravings.

12. **Answer: D.** Nalbuphine

Nalbuphine is an opioid analgesic with κ-agonist/partial μ-antagonistic properties. It does not have a role in the management of opioid overdose. Naloxone, naltrexone, and nalmefene are opioid antagonists that can displace the agonist at opioid receptor and thus used in opioid overdose.

13. **Answer: E.** None of the above

Carbamazepine, chlordiazepoxide, lorazepam, and diazepam can be used to treat alcohol withdrawal syndrome. Carbamazepine is typically used as an adjunctive agent.

14. **Answer: C.** Stimulant withdrawal

Clonidine has a role in the treatment of withdrawal from opioids, alcohol, nicotine, and benzodiazepines. It does not have a role in the treatment of stimulant withdrawal (cocaine and methamphetamine). Trazodone and diphenhydramine are commonly used for sedation in patients undergoing stimulant withdrawal.

15. **Answer: D.** GHB for nonmedical use is a schedule III drug, and when prescribed for medical indications, it is a schedule I substance

GHB sodium is an endogenous compound, and sodium oxybate is the drug name for the identical compound. Illicit GHB is taken at frequent intervals along with other drugs, whereas sodium oxybate is taken at bedtime and not to be taken with alcohol or CNS depressants. Illicit GHB for nonmedical use is a schedule I drug, and when prescribed for medical indications, it is a schedule III substance.

16. **Answer: B.** Acidification of urine

The patient is intoxicated with hallucinogen phencyclidine (PCP). PCP levels are enhanced in acidic urine. Thus, acidification of urine is an adjunct therapy in PCP overdose.

17. **Answer: D.** Acamprosate

Acamprosate and naltrexone are FDA indicated in maintenance of abstinence in alcoholism. However, acamprosate would be a better choice because it is safe to be used in patients with hepatic dysfunction. Naltrexone and disulfiram are not indicated in a patient with hepatic dysfunction. Lorazepam has no role in the management of alcoholism.

18. **Answer: A.** Nortriptyline

Nortriptyline and clonidine are commonly used as second-line agents and are not approved by FDA for the treatment of nicotine dependence.

19. **Answer: B.** Nicotine nasal spray

Among the different nicotine replacement therapy, nicotine nasal spray has the most rapid onset of action (peak action within 1 to 4 minutes), thus providing more immediate relief from cravings. Peak actions with the gum, the inhaler, and the transdermal formulations are 15 to 30 minutes, 15 minutes, and 2 to 4 hours, respectively.

20. **Answer: D.** Methadone has very low risk for abuse

Methadone is contraindicated with ziprasidone and thioridazine because their concurrent use can increase QTc interval and lead to torsades de pointes and sudden death. Methadone can induce its own metabolism and levels vary over time with a 3.5-fold increase in clearance between induction and steady state levels. Methadone is an agonist at the μ-opiate receptor. Although methadone does not provide a quick or potent high, the availability of methadone for treatment and pain has increased its abuse potential.

21. **Answer: B.** Acetaldehyde

Disulfiram irreversibly inhibits the enzyme acetaldehyde dehydrogenase that results in the accumulation of acetaldehyde. Acetaldehyde may cause symptoms such as increased heart rate, hypotension, shortness of breath, nausea, vomiting, headache, confusion, and visual disturbance, after ingestion of alcohol during disulfiram therapy.

22. **Answer: C.** Like naltrexone, acamprosate has been shown to specially reduce heavy drinking

Acamprosate normalizes the dysregulation of N-methyl-D-aspartate (NMDA)-mediated glutamatergic neurotransmission that occurs during early abstinence. Acamprosate should be initiated in patients who are abstinent at treatment. The recommendation is to initiate acamprosate as soon as possible after alcohol withdrawal, when the patient has achieved abstinence. It is contraindicated in severe renal impairment, that is, creatinine clearance of 30 ml per minute or less. Naltrexone has been shown to specially reduce heavy drinking, and acamprosate has been shown to reduce the frequency of drinking. Recommended dose of acamprosate is 660 mg twice a day.

23. **Answer: B.** Oxycodone

Naltrexone produces antagonistic effects by competitively displacing opiate molecules at opiate receptors as well as blocking the access of narcotics to opiate receptor sites. Concurrent administration of naltrexone and opioid analgesics such as oxycodone is contraindicated because naltrexone will reverse the effects of narcotic analgesics resulting in acute withdrawal symptoms. Although tramadol is a centrally acting opioid analgesic that exerts its effect by binding to μ-opioid receptors, there is no drug–drug interaction between naltrexone and tramadol. Hence, tramadol can be safely used for analgesia in patients on naltrexone therapy. There is no drug–drug interaction reported with diazepam, diclofenac sodium, and fluoxetine.

24. **Answer: E.** All of the above

Bupropion is FDA approved for nicotine dependence. It acts by antagonizing nicotinic acetylcholine receptors and inhibiting dopamine and noradrenaline reuptake. Thus, by increasing noradrenaline neurotransmission, bupropion may attenuate nicotine withdrawal symptoms.

25. **Answer: B.** Lorazepam

Benzodiazepines such as diazepam, chlordiazepoxide, and lorazepam are used to prevent delirium tremens. However, diazepam and chlordiazepoxide are not indicated in a patient with liver cirrhosis.

26. **Answer: D.** Naloxone

Naloxone, an opioid antagonist, is approved for management of opioid overdose. Naloxone acts by competing for the μ-, κ-, and σ-opiate receptor sites in the CNS and can displace the agonist at opioid receptor. Flumazenil is used for reversing benzodiazepine activity.

27. **Answer: E.** Stop naltrexone and plan for surgery in 72 hours

Naltrexone should be discontinued 48 to 72 hours before an elective surgery, where opioid analgesia may be required.

28. **Answer: B.** Hydroxyzine

Benzodiazepines should be avoided in a patient with active alcohol use. Hydroxyzine is FDA approved for the treatment of anxiety disorder and may be used on an as-needed basis.

29. **Answer: D.** Metronidazole

Concurrent use of disulfiram and metronidazole is contraindicated. When administered together they may result in CNS toxicity. Psychotic episodes and confusional states have been reported. Metronidazole should not be used in patients who have received disulfiram within the past 14 days. Concurrent use of disulfiram and chlordiazepoxide may increase the serum concentrations of chlordiazepoxide; however, no interactions have been identified with the concurrent use of disulfiram and lorazepam.

30. **Answer: A.** Liver function test (LFT)

LFTs should be closely monitored during naltrexone therapy. Initial screening at baseline and follow-up LFTs should be obtained after 1 month of naltrexone treatment. Follow-up LFTs may then be performed at 3 and 6 months after the initiation of treatment, based on the individual case. Frequent monitoring is indicated when baseline LFT is high or with a history of past hepatic dysfunction.

Chapter 5

Miscellaneous Topics

Questions

1. Which of the following statements is true regarding placebo responders in antidepressant trials?

   A. Placebo responders and antidepressant medication responders have similar changes in brain function after treatment

   B. The placebo response rate in antidepressant studies is around 25%

   C. Early, abrupt, or nonpersistent responses are characteristics of placebo responders

   D. Nonpersistent responders to a drug would have better prognosis

   E. Placebo responders have fewer relapses

2. Which of the following statements best defines phase 3 clinical trials?

   A. The experimental drug is given to a larger group of people to test its effectiveness and to further evaluate its safety

   B. The experimental study drug is tested in large clinical studies to confirm its effectiveness, monitor side effects, compare it with commonly used treatments, and collect information that will allow the drug to be used safely

   C. The experimental drug is tested in a small group of people for the first time to evaluate its safety, determine a safe dosage range, and identify side effects

   D. The experimental drug is administered in a single subtherapeutic dose to a small number of participants to gather preliminary data on the agent's pharmacokinetics and pharmacodynamics

   E. Postmarketing studies that provide additional information including the drug's risks, benefits, and optimal use

3. Which of the following statements regarding the serotonin transporter (SERT) (5-HTT) protein and antidepressant therapy is true?

   A. Individuals with lower 5-HTT expression respond less favorably to antidepressant medications

   B. Individuals with lower 5-HTT are less likely to experience antidepressant-induced side effects

   C. Individuals with lower 5-HTT are more likely to experience antidepressant-induced side effects

   D. Individuals with lower 5-HTT expression are likely to have a rapid response to antidepressant treatment

   E. All of the above

4. Which of the following statements is true regarding the concept of number needed to treat (NNT) in clinical trials?

  A. The NNT is the number of patients who need to be treated to prevent one additional bad outcome

  B. NTT can be calculated as the inverse of the absolute risk reduction (ARR) in randomized control trials

  C. NNT values alone should not be used by providers to communicate risk of an intervention to patients

  D. NNTs calculated from systematic reviews of randomized controlled trials provide the highest level of evidence because systematic reviews contain data from a large number of patients

  E. All of the above

5. Which of the following statements is most accurate regarding the Food and Drug Administration (FDA) requirement for approval of a generic drug?

  A. The FDA requires the generic drug company to submit the results of only one bioequivalence study and not reveal the findings from failed bioequivalence studies

  B. The FDA requires the company to conduct clinical studies of efficacy and safety with the generic drug

  C. The FDA standards for variations in peak plasma concentrations and the total area under the plasma concentration time curve are the same for new branded drugs and generic versions

  D. Generic drugs can have different clinical indications

  E. All of the above

6. In small clinical studies, the glutamatergic system is a promising area of research in mood disorders and likely to offer new possibilities in therapeutics. Which of the following N-methyl-D-aspartate (NMDA) antagonists has been demonstrated to produce antidepressant effects within a few hours of its administration?

    A. Memantine

    B. Intravenous ketamine

    C. Intravenous riluzole

    D. Pramipexole

    E. Intravenous dextromethorphan

7. A 48-year-old man with treatment-resistant depression to multiple antidepressant trials had undergone vagal nerve stimulator implantation 28 months ago. The procedure was well tolerated with no adverse effects. He benefited from improvement in mood and no inpatient admissions. Three days ago, he presented to your clinic with pyrexia, neck stiffness, and photophobia. He was admitted to medical department for meningitis, and his cerebrospinal fluid culture grew pan-sensitive *Staphylococcus aureus*. Which of the following condition would warrant explantation of the vagal nerve stimulator?

    A. Infection refractory to antibiotics

    B. Hardware failure

    C. Potential systemic infection

    D. Need for magnetic resonance imaging (MRI) of the head

    E. All of the above

8. Which of the following is the most common side effect with vagus nerve stimulation (VNS) in the treatment of depression?

    A. Neck pain

    B. Hoarseness

    C. Headache

    D. Cough

    E. Dysesthesia of the throat

9. Which of the following statements is true regarding VNS in the treatment of depression?

    A. The VNS device can be temporarily shut off to permit electroconvulsive therapy (ECT) to be administered

    B. VNS can be particularly useful in treating psychotic depression

    C. MRI of the brain is absolutely contraindicated with VNS implant

    D. VNS is FDA approved for chronic, recurrent unipolar depression and not for bipolar depression

    E. VNS is FDA approved for chronic, recurrent unipolar, or bipolar depression, with at least three failed antidepressant trials

10. Which of the following is true regarding repetitive transcranial magnetic stimulation (TMS)?

    A. Headache is the most common adverse effect

    B. TMS can cause seizure

    C. TMS can temporarily cause aphasia

    D. FDA approved the use of repetitive TMS for treatment of depression in patients, for whom one antidepressant trial at adequate does and duration, failed to respond

    E. All of the above

11. Which of the following drugs is frequently used as anesthetic agent during ECT?

    A. Methohexital

    B. Phenobarbital

    C. Amobarbital

    D. Paraldehyde

    E. Nitrous oxide

12. Which of the following conditions may respond well to ECT?

    A. Parkinson disease

    B. Intractable seizures

    C. Catatonia

    D. Neuroleptic malignant syndrome

    E. All of the above

13. All of the following are true regarding TMS EXCEPT:

    A. Creates a powerful electrical current near the scalp

    B. Coil on the scalp creates a potent magnetic field

    C. Electrodeless magnetic stimulation

    D. It is a FDA-approved antidepressant treatment

    E. None of the above

14. Which of the following advantages does ultrabrief ECT offer over conventional brief ECT?

    A. Ultrabrief ECT produces less retrograde amnesia

    B. Ultrabrief ECT delivers less total current to the brain

    C. Ultrabrief ECT uses short-duration square wave electrical pulses

    D. Ultrabrief ECT in bipolar depression patients may have a more rapid response than patients with unipolar depression

    E. All of the above

15. The anesthetic agent propofol has been shown to have lesser cardio-vascular effects than methohexital and can be used in patients with preexisting cardiac conditions during ECT. Which of the following is a drawback of using propofol during ECT?

    A. Higher incidence of post-ECT delirium

    B. Shortening of the seizure length

    C. Postictal agitation

    D. Cost of the drug

    E. All of the above

16. TMS is reported to be effective in which of the following conditions?

    A. Depression

    B. Obsessive–compulsive disorder (OCD)

    C. Acute and chronic pain

    D. Posttraumatic stress disorder

    E. All of the above

17. All of the following herbs have been implicated with psychotic symptoms EXCEPT:

    A. *Cinnamomum camphora*

    B. Passion flower

    C. Yangjinhua

    D. Kava-kava

    E. Mormon tea

18. Concurrent administration of which of the following medications can increase the risk of neurotoxicity during ECT therapy?

    A. Lithium

    B. Valproate

    C. Lamotrigine

    D. Aripiprazole

    E. Venlafaxine

19. ECT has a role in the management of all of the following conditions EXCEPT:

    A. Prior good response to ECT

    B. Risk of suicide

    C. Serotonin syndrome

    D. Treatment-resistant depression

    E. None of the above

Answers

1. **Answer: C.** Early, abrupt, or nonpersistent responses are characteristics of placebo responders

The rate of placebo responders in antidepressant trials ranges between 25% and 60%. Early, abrupt, or nonpersistent responses are characteristics of placebo responders. They have the worst prognosis and a higher number of relapses compared with persistent responders.

2. **Answer: B.** The experimental study drug is tested in large clinical studies to confirm its effectiveness, monitor side effects, compare it with commonly used treatments, and collect information that will allow the drug to be used safely

Clinical trials are classified into four phases. Phase I are designed to assess the safety, pharmacokinetics, and pharmacodynamics of an investigational new drug. Phase II assesses dosing requirements (phase II A) and efficacy (phase II B). Phase III aims at testing the new drug in large clinical studies to confirm its effectiveness, monitor side effects, compare it with commonly used treatments, and collect information that will allow the drug to be used safely. Phase IV involves postmarketing studies that provide additional information including the drug's risks, benefits, and optimal use. Phase 0 is the first-in-human trial where the experimental drug is administered in a single subtherapeutic dose to a small number of participants to gather preliminary data on the agent's pharmacokinetics and pharmacodynamics.

3. **Answer: A.** Individuals with lower 5-HTT expression respond less favorably to antidepressant medications

The SERT plays an important role in reuptake and release of serotonin from the neurons. SSRIs target SERT to block uptake of serotonin and improve serotonin neurotransmission. The short allele of SERT gene polymorphism 5-HTTLPR is associated with lower expression of SERT. Lower expression of SERT is negatively associated with SSRI therapy. Thus, SSRIs work less favorably in individuals carrying short allele of SERT gene polymorphism.

4. **Answer: E.** All of the above

The NNT is the number of patients you need to treat to prevent one additional adverse outcome. It is the inverse of ARR. Health care providers should not communicate the risk of intervention to the patients based on NNTs. NNTs calculated from systematic reviews of randomized controlled trials provide the highest level of evidence because systematic reviews contain data from a large group of patients.

5. **Answer: A.** The FDA requires the generic drug company to submit the results of only one bioequivalence study and not reveal the findings from failed bioequivalence studies

The FDA does not require generic manufacturers to conduct clinical studies of efficacy and safety with the generic drug because these trials have been conducted by the brand name company. The FDA requires the generic drug company to submit the results of only one bioequivalence study and not reveal the findings from failed bioequivalence studies.

6. **Answer: B.** Intravenous ketamine

Ketamine, an NMDA antagonist, has been demonstrated to produce antidepressant effects within a few hours of its administration. The glutamatergic system is a promising area of research in mood disorders and is likely to offer new possibilities in therapeutics.

7. **Answer: E.** All of the above

Vagal nerve stimulation is an option for the treatment of chronic refractory depression. Device removal is indicated in infection as, in this case, insufficient clinical response, severe side effects, surgical complications such as hardware failure, or when MRI/radiotherapy is needed.

8. **Answer: B.** Hoarseness

The most common side effect with VNS in the treatment of depression is hoarseness. VNS is typically set at the frequency of 30 seconds of stimulation followed by 5 minutes with no stimulation. Hoarseness of voice is seen during the stimulation phase.

9. **Answer: A.** The VNS device can be temporarily shut off to permit electroconvulsive therapy (ECT) to be administered

VNS was approved by the FDA for the treatment of severe, recurrent unipolar and bipolar depression with a history of at least four failed antidepressant trials. It is not indicated in psychotic depression. The VNS device can be temporarily shut off to permit ECT to be administered. Special precautions need to be taken before obtaining MRI. With special send–receive coils, it is possible to get an MRI of the brain when absolutely indicated.

10. **Answer: E.** All of the above

Headache is the most common adverse effect of repetitive TMS. It can cause seizure and temporarily cause aphasia. The FDA approved the use of repetitive TMS for treatment of depression in patients who failed to respond to one antidepressant trial at adequate dose and duration.

11. **Answer: A.** Methohexital

Methohexital, with its duration of action of about 5 minutes, is an excellent anesthetic agent for ECT. Phenobarbital—a longer acting barbiturate, amobarbital—a shorter acting barbiturate, and paraldehyde—a nonbarbiturate hypnotic are not anesthetic agents. Nitrous oxide is being studied as a substitute for ECT, not as an anesthetic agent in ECT. Nitrous oxide produces a central sympathetic stimulation similar to ECT, releasing endogenous opioid peptides. Nitrous oxide is also associated with seizure-like activity itself.

12. **Answer: E.** All of the above

ECT has a role in the management of Parkinson disease, intractable seizures, catatonia, and neuroleptic malignant syndrome.

13. **Answer: C.** Electrodeless magnetic stimulation

TMS creates a powerful electrical current near the scalp. The coil on the scalp creates a potent magnetic field that is referred as electrodeless electrical stimulation. TMS is approved by FDA as an antidepressant treatment.

14. **Answer: E.** All of the above

Ultrabrief ECT delivers less total current to the brain and thus produces less retrograde amnesia. It uses short-duration square wave electrical pulses. Ultrabrief ECT in bipolar depression patients may have a more rapid response than in patients with unipolar depression.

15. **Answer: B.** Shortening of the seizure length

Propofol is associated with shortening of the seizure length during ECT.

16. **Answer: E.** All of the above

TMS is approved by FDA as an antidepressant treatment. Many studies have shown promising results in using TMS to treat OCD. Literature supports that TMS can acutely decrease pain in healthy adults or patients with chronic pain and posttraumatic stress disorder (PTSD).

17. **Answer: C.** Yangjinhua

Yangjinhua, a Chinese herbal medicine, is used in the treatment of asthma, bronchitis, and pain symptoms and does not cause psychotic symptoms. *C. camphora* (used in inflammatory diseases such as rheumatism, bronchitis, and sprains), mormon tea (used for cold symptoms), passion flower, and kava-kava (used for anxiety) can cause psychotic symptoms.

18. **Answer: A.** Lithium

Lithium is known to increase the neurotoxicity during ECT. Lithium is generally withheld 36 to 48 hours before ECT to avoid delirium, to avoid prolonged seizure, and to reduce the risk of arrhythmia.

19. **Answer: C.** Serotonin syndrome

Elecroconvulsive therapy has a role in the management of patients with a history of prior good response to ECT, treatment-resistant depression, and when rapid response is required such as suicide risk. It has no role in the treatment of serotonin syndrome.

Index